AF413032

....

Psychotropic Drug Use in the Medically Ill

Advances in Psychosomatic Medicine

Vol. 21

Series Editor	*Thomas N. Wise*, Falls Church, Va.
Editors	*G. A. Fava*, Bologna *H. Freyberger*, Hannover *F. Guggenheim*, Little Rock, Ark. *M. Hale*, New Britain, Conn. *O. W. Hill*, London *Z. J. Lipowski*, Toronto, Ont. *G. Lloyd*, London *A. Reading*, Tampa, Fla. *P. Reich*, Boston, Mass. *M. B. Rosenthal*, Cleveland, Ohio
Consulting Editors	*G. L. Engel*, Rochester, N.Y. *H. Weiner*, Los Angeles, Calif. *L. Levi*, Stockholm
Editor Emeritus	*Franz Reichsman*, Brooklyn, N.Y.

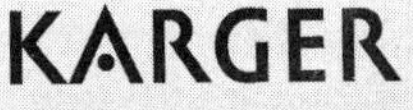

Basel · Freiburg · Paris · London · New York ·
New Delhi · Bangkok · Singapore · Tokyo · Sydney

Psychotropic Drug Use in the Medically Ill

Volume Editor *Paul A. Silver,* Washington, D. C.

1 figure and 8 tables, 1994

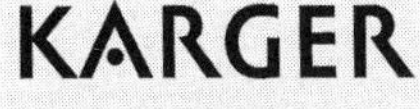

Basel · Freiburg · Paris · London · New York ·
New Delhi · Bangkok · Singapore · Tokyo · Sydney

QV
77
P9775
1994

···························

Advances in Psychosomatic Medicine

Library of Congress Cataloging-in-Publication Data
Psychotropic drug use in the medically ill / volume editor, Paul A. Silver.
(Advances in psychosomatic medicine; vol. 21)
Includes bibliographical references and index. (alk. paper)
1. Psychopharmacology.   2. Psychological manifestations of general diseases – Treatment.
3. Psychotropic drugs.   I. Silver, Paul A., 1953 – .   II. Series.
[DNLM: 1. Psychotropic Drugs – therapeutic use.   2. Psychotropic Drugs – pharmacology.   3. Disease.
W1 AD81 v. 21 1994 / QV 77P9747 1994]
RM 315.P784   1994   615'.788 – dc20
ISBN 3–8055–5969–0

Bibliographic Indices. This publication is listed in bibliographic services, including Current Contents® and Index Medicus

Drug Dosage. The authors and the publisher have exerted every effort to ensure that drug selection and dosage set forth in this text are in accord with current recommendations and practice at the time of publication. However, in view of ongoing research, changes in government regulations, and the constant flow of information relating to drug therapy and drug reactions, the reader is urged to check the package insert for each drug for any change in indications and dosage and for added warnings and precautions. This is particularly important when the recommended agent is a new and/or infrequently employed drug.

All rights reserved. No part of this publication may be translated into other languages, reproduced or utilized in any form or by any means, electronic or mechanical, including photocopying, recording, microcopying, or by any information storage and retrieval system, without permission in writing from the publisher.

© Copyright 1994 by S. Karger AG, P. O. Box, CH–4009 Basel (Switzerland)
Printed in Switzerland on acid-free paper by Thür AG Offsetdruck, Pratteln
ISBN 3–8055–5969–0

Contents

....

Preface

The past two decades have seen a remarkable coalescence of the fields of psychiatry, medicine and neurology. The growth of consultation liaison services, medical psychiatric units and the fields of behavioral neurology, neuropsychiatry and behavioral medicine are indicators of this striving for synthesis. At the same time, the advances in biological psychiatry and psychopharmacology have increased the utilization of somatic interventions in all areas of psychiatry. These parallel developments have resulted in more attention being paid to the pharmacologic treatment of the psychiatric manifestations of nonpsychiatric illnesses as well as the expanding use of somatic treatment in psychiatric patients with comorbid medical conditions. Nonpsychiatric physicians from virtually all clinical fields will have occasion to use psychotropic medications in their patients. Similarly, as the field of psychiatry 'remedicalizes', the bulk of psychiatrists will provide psychopharmacologic treatment to patients with medical conditions. Psychotropic drug use in the medically ill can be exceedingly intricate given the diverse pharmacologic effects of most psychotropic agents and their propensity for interacting with other medications. It is our hope that this edition of *Advances in Psychosomatic Medicine* will be of assistance to all of us who care for these complicated patients.

During the planning of this volume, it was decided to provide in-depth reviews of a limited number of topics rather than attempt to superficially survey the whole field. The contributing authors are clinicians and researchers with profound expertise in their areas. In addition, each paper can, by and large, stand on its own, thus allowing the reader to comprehensively cover a particular subject in a single article. This, by necessity, has led to some between-article repetition. On the whole, the benefits of these approaches should outweigh their shortcomings. With two exceptions, each paper will cover a particular disease process or organ system. The exceptions are Rubey and Lydiard's overview of basic pharmacologic issues in medicating the medically ill and DasGupta and Jefferson's paper on the treatment of mania in the face of medical comorbidity.

The hard work of the contributing authors has produced a work which is, we hope, both scholarly and useful.

Paul A. Silver

Silver PA (ed): Psychotropic Drug Use in the Medically Ill.
Adv Psychosom Med. Basel, Karger, 1994, vol 21, pp 1–27

Psychopharmacology in the Medically Ill

General Principles

Robert N. Rubey, R. Bruce Lydiard

Institute of Psychiatry, Medical University of South Carolina,
Charleston, S. C., USA

The purpose of all drug therapy is clinical efficacy. As a practical matter, this requires the delivery of the right drug to the right place in the right concentration for the right amount of time. Most guidelines available to the clinician for the psychopharmacologic management of psychiatric patients are derived from studies of medically well patient populations; these guidelines may not be reliable for the individual patient in whom pharmacokinetic changes are large enough to require alterations in drug dosages. One factor among many that may produce these pharmacokinetic changes is medical illness.

The purpose of this paper is to review our current understanding of how psychopharmacologic agents are to be used in medically ill patients, as well as to review the pharmacokinetic and pharmacodynamic changes that occur in these patients as a result of disease processes. This topic is vast, and cannot be completely covered here; we have chosen to confine our discussion to psychopharmacology in patients with impaired function of liver, kidney, or lung, with the hope that this will apply to a large percentage of medically ill patients commonly seen in clinical practice. Psychopharmacology in patients with impaired cardiac function is dealt with in a separate paper in this volume.

This paper is divided into four sections. In the first section some general principles of psychopharmacology in normal individuals without medical illness are reviewed, including an overview of basic pharmacodynamics and pharmacokinetics, as well as a brief review of amine receptors. The remaining three sections deal, respectively, with psychopharmacologic treatment of patients with liver, kidney, or lung disease.

General Principles

Pharmacodynamics

Pharmacodynamics is the relationship between drug concentration and drug effect. In general, drug effect rises as a function of drug concentration until some maximal effect is achieved, beyond which increasing drug concentration produces no additional (beneficial) effect. Drugs vary with respect to maximal effect, and are therefore said to vary in efficacy. Drug potency is the effect that a drug has at any given concentration. Drugs may (and usually do) differ with respect to potency, but may be equally efficacious. For example, it is generally true that all neuroleptics have equal efficacy with respect to their antipsychotic effects, but differ widely with respect to their potency.

Pharmacologic agents that have only one effect are seldom encountered in psychopharmacology. 'Side effects' are in reality additional (and usually unwanted) effects of drug action, and each effect has its own equation for 'efficacy' and 'potency'. For a drug to be tolerable in any given patient, efficacy must occur at a drug concentration below the concentration that is associated with unacceptable subjective and physiologic side effects.

In psychopharmacology, the relationship between 'concentration' and 'effect' is described by the neurotransmitter/receptor model. This subject is extremely complex and incompletely understood. In the most basic terms, it is believed that communication among neurons is mediated through various classes of neurotransmitters acting at specific receptor sites. In most cases, the desired therapeutic effect occurs days or even weeks after sufficient drug concentration has been achieved, leading to the hypothesis that neurotransmitter/receptor interaction is not in itself a sufficient explanation for the effect. Rather, it is now believed that the effect may in some way be involved with changes in receptor function, reflected in altered receptor density and/or altered sensitivity of the receptor itself.

As mentioned above, most psychopharmacologic agents have not only their desired (therapeutic) effects, but side effects as well. This multiplicity of effect may be explained in a number of ways, including the presence of specific receptors in different parts of the central nervous system, each subserving a different function. For example, it is believed that the antipsychotic effect of the various neuroleptics is achieved by blockade of D-2 receptors in the forebrain, while concurrent blockade of the same receptors in the striatum leads to the extrapyramidal side effects caused by the same drugs. In the case of the antidepressants, many agents are believed to have their therapeutic effect (alleviation of depression) by blocking the reuptake of neurotransmitter into the presynaptic neuron, thereby increasing the availability of the transmitter at the synaptic cleft. However, increased serotonin availability may lead not only to alleviation of depression, but also to gastrointestinal distress, anorexia, sexual dysfunction as well as other effects attributable to manipulation of the serotonin system. These 'side effects' usually occur before the antidepressant effect.

Other antidepressants are thought to have their therapeutic effect through blockade of norepinephrine reuptake; however, increased norepinephrine availability may also result in tremors, tachycardia, and sexual dysfunction. Blockade of dopamine uptake and increased dopamine availability may lead to aggravation of psychosis.

Side effects of psychopharmacologic agents may be due not only to reuptake blockade leading to increased synaptic availability of norepinephrine, serotonin, or dopamine, but also to concurrent direct antagonist activity at other receptors as well. For example, antagonist activity at the muscarinic receptor (one of two known classes of acetylcholine receptor) by neuroleptics and tricyclics may cause blurred vision, tachycardia, urinary retention, dry mouth, impaired memory, and constipation. Antagonist activity at the H1 (histamine) receptor may cause sedation and weight gain, while activity at the alpha-1 (adrenergic) receptor may cause postural hypotension and sedation.

According to the transmitter/receptor model, the proximate cause of drug effect(s) is concentration of drug at the receptor. However, clinicians are not able to inject drug directly into the synaptic cleft, and so must rely on the body itself to deliver the drug from the site of administration (by mouth, by direct injection into tissue or vein, or by transdermal absorption) to the site of action. In this process the body may alter the drug in many ways, and the sum of these actions by the body on the drug are called the pharmacokinetics of the drug.

Pharmacokinetics

For the purpose of pharmacokinetic description, the passage of a drug from the point of its absorption to its ultimate biotransformation or excretion is broken into four stages: absorption, distribution, metabolism, and excretion. There is wide interindividual pharmacokinetic variation with respect to each of these phases, so that a given dosage of a drug may lead to very different drug concentrations from individual to individual. In addition, there may be great intraindividual variation as well: the indiviudal's age, health, metabolic and nutritional states will all change over time, and these changes, as well as a multitude of other factors, will all affect drug pharmacokinetics.

A detailed description of pharmacokinetics is beyond the scope of this paper. However, a few terms that will be encountered later in the paper will be briefly discussed here. Volume of distribution is a term used to describe pharmacokinetics during the distribution phase. In essence, volume of distribution is a way of conceptualizing how widely in the body a particular drug is distributed, and to explain why a given dosage of one drug will result in a high serum level of that drug, while the same dosage of another drug results in a low serum level. In mathematical terms, it is the dosage of drug administered divided by serum concentration (both bound and unbound fractions). Drugs which are highly bound to serum proteins and stay within the vascular compartment will tend to have a low volume of distribution, while those which more readily pass out of the vascular compartment will have higher volumes of distribution.

Drug half-life is defined as the time that it takes for the body to eliminate, whether by direct excretion or by metabolism, one-half of the amount of that drug in the body. Most psychopharmacologic agents follow first-order kinetics, so that a constant percentage (rather than a constant amount) of drug is eliminated per unit time. In other words, it takes as long for the concentration of a hypothetical drug to go from 100 to 50 mg as it does to go from 50 to 25 mg, although the absolute quantity of drug eliminated is twice as great in the first interval than in the second. At a constant dosing schedule, drug steady state will occur when the amount cleared as equal to the amount administered; this will occur at between 5 and 7 half-lives of the particular drug being administered.

Clearance is a rate term, and refers to the volume of serum from which a particular drug is completely and irreversibly removed per unit time. In general, this occurs either by drug metabolism (inactivation), excretion, or a combination of both. Clearance is the rate of drug elimination, and is a measure of the efficiency of all metabolic and excretory activities, primarily occurring in the liver and kidney.

To summarize: half-life is the amount of time required to remove one-half of the total amount of a particular drug from the body; volume of distribution is the volume into which a particular drug distributes; and clearance is the rate at which a given volume of blood is irreversibly cleared of drug. Accordingly, half-life will vary directly with volume of distribution and inversely with clearance in the following way:

$$t^{1/2} = k \text{ (volume of distribution/clearance)},$$

where k is a constant equal to the natural log of $1/2$ or 0.693.

It is important to remember that all psychotropics except lithium are protein bound to one degree or another, and that more highly bound drugs distribute less widely (have smaller volumes of distribution) and are eliminated more slowly than drugs that are less protein bound. Therefore, conditions that affect degree of protein binding will also affect volume of distribution, clearance, and half-life. These conditions include (among others) medical illness, nutritional status, age, and competition from other protein-bound drugs, and will be discussed in more detail in subsequent sections of this paper. For example, liver disease often results in decreased protein production with subsequent increased free fraction of any drug that is bound; the implications of this event are discussed in the next section.

Psychopharmacology in Patients with Impaired Liver Function

With the notable exception of lithium, most psychopharmacologic agents are metabolized by the liver. It follows from this that knowledge of the effects of liver disease on the absorption, distribution, metabolism, and elimination of psychotropic medications is of particular importance to clinicians prescribing these agents. Various attempts have made to find a liver function test, or combination of tests, that would define liver function in the way serum creatinine, blood urea nitrogen, and creatinine clearance define kidney function, and thereby provide a guide to pharmacologic management; with few exceptions [1], researchers in this area have not been encouraged by the results [2–5].

This said, most authors would agree that of all patients with liver disease, cirrhotics are most at risk for side effects from medication; and there is also evidence that those with encephalopathy, whether past or current, may be at increased risk [6]. Apart from cirrhosis, however, the picture is quite variable: in acute viral hepatitis, for example, clearance of some drugs is decreased (half-life prolonged), while for others there is no change from normal age-matched controls. Further complicating the picture, liver disease usually cannot be considered by itself alone. Very often drug metabolites, the products of liver metabolism, are excreted by the kidney as well as in the bile, and these metabolites may be pharmacologically active. In consequence, renal function must also often be considered when adjusting dosages and dosing schedules. Finally, most psychotropics are protein bound, and liver disease, especially chronic disease, results in decreased protein production; this often results in an increased free fraction of drug [7].

Normal Liver Function in Drug Metabolism and Elimination

Hepatic metabolism is determined by hepatic blood flow, degree of enzymatic capacity in the parenchyma, and degree of protein binding of a particular agent. In general terms, the liver alters lipophilic drugs so that they become more water soluble, and can be more efficiently removed from blood by the kidney. This biotransformation may occur in two phases: the first phase is oxidative, reductive, or hydrolytic. The most important oxidative enzyme system is the cytochrome P-450 system, located primarily in the hepatic smooth endoplasmic reticulum. This location is important because it makes the enzyme system highly accessible to lipophilic compounds. The activity of this and other microsomal systems shows great inter-individual variations, and metabolic rates may vary by a factor of six or more from person to person [8]. In the second phase of biotransformation, the metabolites of the first phase may be conjugated with sugars, sulfates, or amino acids, again rendering a more hydrophilic compound; this also occurs largely in the hepatic smooth endoplasmic reticulum.

Some drugs may act to increase the synthesis of the cytochrome P-450 system enzymes, thereby increasing rates of drug metabolism and subsequent elimination. Examples of such drugs include alcohol, chloral hydrate, carbamazepine, phenobarbital, phenytoin, as well as many others [9, p. 85]. Some drugs may inhibit hepatic enzyme activity, including MAO inhibitors, methylphenidate, and others [9, p. 87].

Alterations in Liver Function in Disease States

Liver function may be compromised by infection, neoplasms, or toxic insult. Damage may vary from slight to severe, and may affect the intrinsic metabolic activity of liver enzymes, or the architecture of the liver itself, or both. The liver has considerable reserve capacity as well as regenerative potential, so that some disease states may not cause any clinically significant alteration in liver function. In other instances, such as acute viral hepatitis, liver function may be compromised to a clinically significant degree during the active phase of the illness, but return to normal as the infection clears. Chronic liver disease, however, may deplete hepatic reserves to the point where drug metabolism, binding, and distribution may be affected.

If the specific disease process is chronic or unremitting, or if the exposure to toxic chemicals (especially alcohol) overwhelms the liver's regenerative capacity, normal liver architecture may be disrupted. Cirrhosis is the classic example of this process, and results from the formation of collagen into connective tissue scars. It follows from this that normal blood flow through the liver is disrupted, and, as pressure in the portal venous system builds, collateral channels carry more of the flow, bypassing the liver and decreasing the amount of drug exposed to first-pass metabolism. Neoplasms may have similar effects on hepatic architecture, although there is great variability in this process, varying with tumor size and type, as well as many other factors. At the cellular level, less total flow is available to hepatocytes for metabolic processing; individual hepatocytes become more isolated from the flow that is available, and cytochrome P-450 enzyme activity decreases too. The end result of these processes is reduced intrinsic metabolism by the liver.

As mentioned above, volume of distribution is defined as administered dose divided by serum concentration of bound and unbound fractions; it is a measure of how widely a particular drug distributes in the body. Lipid-soluble drugs distribute widely, and have large volumes of distribution, while water-soluble drugs do not distribute as widely, and have smaller volumes of distribution.

Volume of distribution varies with age, weight, and sex, as well as an disease processes. Hepatic disease may increase the volume of distribution in several significant ways: first, decreased protein production, especially albumin, makes more unbound drug available for distribution into the tissue compartment; second, decreased intrinsic metabolism of lipid-soluble drugs to more hydrophilic compounds also increases the fraction of drug available for distribution into the intracellular compartment; third, ascites may develop as a result of liver disease, which increases total body water; and, fourth, elevated serum bilirubin competes with unbound drug for protein binding sites, further increasing the unbound fraction of drug.

An increase in volume of distribution does not necessarily lead to increased drug half-life. Half-life is directly related to volume of distribution but is inversely related to clearance, which is a rate term, describing the amount of serum cleared of drug per unit time. Half-life increases as clearance decreases. Clearance is the rate of elimination; it is a measure of the efficiency of the sum of all metabolic and excretory activities, primarily occurring in the liver and kidney. In disease states, intrinsic metabolic activity in the liver both increases (due to increased unbound fraction of drug available for metabolism) and decreases (due to decreased enzyme activity and poor parenchymal microcirculation); the net effect, however, is decreased drug metabolism, becoming clinically significant when activity drops beneath the reserve capacity of the organ.

The excretory activity of the kidney may actually increase in disease states, so long as kidney function remains within normal limits: bound drug is not filtered by the kidney glomerulus, but unbound drug is freely filtered. As the unbound fraction rises as a result of impaired liver function, the rate of drug elimination by the kidney increases.

To summarize, the effects of liver disease states on drug volume of distribution and metabolism, and therefore on drug half-life, are complex and overlapping. In a broad sense, the interactions among three main factors must be considered: intrinsic metabolic activity, free fraction of drug, and effective hepatic blood flow. Disease states affect each of these factors differently and to different degrees, and each drug differs from other drugs in its sensitivity to alterations in metabolic activity or changes in blood flow. For example, nortriptyline is more highly extracted by the liver than diazepam, so that nortriptyline elimination is more sensitive to changes in flow than is diazepam, which is by contrast more sensitive to declines in intrinsic metabolic activity [10].

As noted above, if the effects of disease on the intrinsic metabolic activity of the liver are considered, two broad and opposing forces emerge: on the one hand, intrinsic metabolic activity will decline with hepatocellular death and with disruptions of hepatic architecture; on the other hand, metabolic activity will increase as more free (unbound) drug is available to be cleared by the remaining hepatocytes. The net effect will depend on which factor is predominant at any particular stage of the disease, so that clearance may be unchanged, decreased, or even increased [11].

Some drugs are known to induce hepatic microsomal enzyme activity in the normal liver, and these drugs may actually serve to maintain enzymatic activity for a time in the failing liver; other drugs are known to inhibit enzyme activity, and will have the opposite effect. As disease progresses, however, negative forces will predominate, hepatic metabolism will fall, clearance will decline, and drug half-life as a function of clearance will be prolonged.

In chronic disease states, especially cirrhosis, all three factors described above are affected: intrinsic metabolic activity is diminished, hepatic architecture and blood flow are disrupted, and protein binding (due to diminished protein production and high protein content in ascitic fluid) declines. With respect to intrinsic metabolic activity, however, it has been repeatedly observed that drugs undergoing extensive oxidative metabolism (such as diazepam) are more significantly affected than those undergoing primarily conjugative metabolism (such as lorazepam, temazepam, and oxazepam) [12–14]. The reason for this is not well understood, but as a result, highly protein bound and highly extracted drugs that undergo oxidative metabolism will have greater unbound fractions and extended half-lives in cirrhotic patients when compared to normals.

Cirrhosis is a chronic process; in patients with acute illness, it may be said in general that most drug metabolism is not altered in mild-to-moderate disease. However, in cases of severe viral hepatitis, as in cirrhosis, drugs that undergo extensive oxidative metabolism may have greater unbound fractions and extended half-lives [15, 16].

Finally, it should be remembered that patients with severe liver disease, especially cirrhosis, may develop the hepatorenal syndrome, with decreasing glomerular filtration rates, oliguria, and poor renal indices. The syndrome is almost always accompanied by ascites as well as other signs of liver failure, and may progress to complete renal failure [17]. As many psychotropic medications have active metabolites, and these metabolites may be excreted by the kidneys, dosages will have to be adjusted in these patients.

Clinical Considerations

No reliable noninvasive test or combination of tests have yet been found to be consistent guides to the clinician in the administration of psychotropic medications to patients with liver disease; specifically, no measure comparable to glomerular filtration rate in kidney disease has been found for liver disease. Almost all psychopharmacologic agents are metabolized primarily by the liver; it would follow from this that these medications are especially problematic in patients with impaired liver disease, and that care should be taken to reduce dosages of these medications in such patients. While this is undoubtedly true, studies have not shown that, in general, medications cleared primarily by the liver are most liable to give adverse effects in liver disease [18].

Specific Guidelines

Although it is difficult to give specific guidelines for dosage adjustments, the following suggestions may be offered on dosing the most commonly used classes of psychotropic drugs.

Benzodiazepines

There have been occasional case reports of direct hepatotoxicity from the use of diazepam [19] and alprazolam [20]. Benzodiazepines have been well studied in cirrhotic patients, and with somewhat varied results; in general there is agreement that the benzodiazepines that are metabolized primarily by conjugation rather than oxidation, specifically lorazepam, temazepam, and oxazepam, are best tolerated [6, 12, 13, 21–25]. If a benzodiazepine other than one of these is desirable in a specific patient, it would be wise to decrease dosage by one-half in patients with severe liver disease [26]. Sedation in patients with liver disease seems to be especially a problem in patients whose disease is secondary to alcoholism, and to those with a history of encephalopathy [6, 18].

Neuroleptics

Rare cases of clinical jaundice and cholestatic hepatitis have been reported with all classes of the phenothiazines, and most often with chlorpromazine, although this may have more to do with the frequency with which it has been used. The incidence of chlorpromazine-related jaundice in eight studies reviewed by Ishak and Irey [27] was estimated to be 1.2%. Haloperidol-related cases have also been reported [28], while thioxanthene-related cases have not. The mechanism for this apparent direct hepatotoxicity is not clear;

there are suggestions that both immunologic/hypersensitivity, as well as cytotoxic mechanisms, may be involved [29].

When neuroleptics are given to patients with preexisting liver disease,
greatly elevated serum levels may result [30]. Phenothiazines (i.e. chlorpromazine, thioridazine, fluphenazine, perphenazine, and trifluoperazine, among
others) should be avoided where possible, and should not be given when patients have cholestatic jaundice. In addition, a history of encephalopathy may
also argue against the use of chlorpromazine: Read et al. [31] found that chlorpromazine given orally in a dose of 1 mg/kg in patients with cirrhosis and a history of encephalopathy caused abnormal slowing of the EEG, suggesting an
increased sensitivity to this drug.

Dosages of all neuroleptics should be reduced when these drugs are given
to patients with liver disease, and levels monitored when possible. If the general guidelines of Arns et al. [10] (tab. 1) are followed, the reductions should
be by at least 25%. Haloperidol may be the best choice in this patient population: it has only one potentially important metabolite, and serum levels for the
parent compound may be followed and adjusted to fall in the usually effective
range of 5–30 ng/ml. In addition, liver enzymes should be followed for the first
2 months of therapy [32].

Antidepressants

Relatively few data are available on the effects of liver disease on the
pharmacokinetics of antidepressants, although these effects could be significant. The antidepressants as a class are highly protein bound, and the unbound
fraction of these drugs will rise in patients with liver disease. In addition, the
antidepressants are highly extracted by the liver in first-pass metabolism; as
liver disease progresses, the fraction extracted will fall due to decreased liver
perfusion and decreased intrinsic enzymatic metabolism. This will be true for
both the TCAs and for the newer antidepressants; however, because 50% or
more of cirrhotic patients may have latent or subclinical encephalopathy [33],
it is probably advisable to choose nonsedating drugs. As a class, the SSRIs (fluoxetine, sertraline, and paroxetine) are less sedating than the TCAs, and therefore may be preferable in these patients. It is important to emphasize, however, that the newer antidepressants, including both the SSRIs and bupropion,
are not as yet extensively studied in patients with chronic liver disease.

Fluoxetine and bupropion are highly protein bound and subject to extensive first-pass metabolism; both have pharmacologically active metabolites, although in the case of bupropion its major metabolite may actually be antago-
nistic to the parent drug [34]. Schenker et al. [35] studied the use of fluoxetine
in 14 patients with well-compensated cirrhosis and without ascites or significant protein deficits. Their data show a tripling of $t\frac{1}{2}$ from a mean of 2.2 to

6.6 days for the parent compound, as well as accumulation of the desmethyl metabolite, which has an even longer half-life. They recommend a dosage reduction of 50% in this population, and suggest that even greater reductions might be indicated for patients with more severe disease. A study by Devane et al. [36] on clearance of bupropion and its metabolites after a single dose given to 8 volunteers, 5 of whom had cirrhosis, found an increased half-life for one metabolite but no significant change in half-life for the parent drug or its other metabolites. The authors point out the need for caution in interpretation of these findings, especially when consideration is being given to using a drug which has proven epileptigenic properties in a population which includes a high percentage of alcoholics.

In an uncontrolled study, Krastev et al. [37] studied the effects of a single dose of paroxetine in a group of cirrhotic patients and found that plasma concentrations of paroxetine in these patients after 5 days were similar to those obtained from healthy subjects during previous studies. However, when Dalhoff et al. [38] conducted a controlled study of cirrhotics and healthy patients given paroxetine 20–30 mg daily over a 2-week period, they found that in the cirrhotic patients plasma concentrations were higher and half-lives increased.

There are no published data on the use of sertraline in this patient population. Sertraline is metabolized extensively in the liver, and its primary metabolite (desmethylsertraline) has a half-life of approximately 60 h in normal subjects. The drug manufacturer recommends caution when using sertraline in patients with significantly impaired liver function.

The MAO inhibitors, phenelzine, isocarboxazide, and tranylcypromine, have been associated with a low incidence of altered liver function or jaundice in normal subjects, and the manufacturers of these drugs recommend that they not be given to patients with liver disease. Moclobemide, a new reversible MAO-A inhibitor, has been studied in cirrhotic patients, and impaired elimination and increased half-life have been found [39].

When the TCAs are used in patients with impaired liver function, dosages should be lowered and serum drug levels followed. Precise guidelines are not currently available; under the format suggested by Arns et al. [10], the antidepressants would fall into the category where decreases of 25% or more are recommended. With respect to drug levels, allowance must be made for the increased unbound fraction that will occur in the context of liver disease; again, precise guidelines are not available and attention to side effects and clinical response must be the rule.

Anticonvulsants
Carbamazepine and valproic acid are both highly protein-bound and almost entirely metabolized in the liver. There appear to be no data on the spe-

Table 1. Modification of drug dosages in hepatic disease[1]

Recommended change in drug dose	Necessary condition
1 No change or minor change	1 Mild liver disease 2 Extensive elimination of drug by kidneys and renal function intact 3 Drug is enzyme limited and given acutely
2 Decrease dose up to 25%	1 Elimination by the liver does not exceed 40%; no renal dysfunction 2 Drug is flow/enyzme limited and given acutely
3 Decrease dose by more than 25%	1 Drug is enzyme limited and given chronically 2 Protein binding is significantly altered 3 Drug is eliminated by the kidneys and renal function is severely affected 4 Altered sensitivity to drug due to liver disease

[1] Adapted from Arns et al. [10].

cific effects of liver disease on carbamazepine elimination; it is reasonable to assume that half-life will increase and clearance will decrease, requiring a reduction of dosage. Blood levels and complete blood counts are essential; the unbound fraction can be expected to increase in the context of liver disease. The use of valproic acid in this population should be avoided, as it has been shown to be directly hepatotoxic and has been associated with rare cases of hepatitis [40]. If it must be used, dosage should be decreased [10], liver function tests monitored, and levels closely followed.

Lithium

Lithium is excreted almost entirely by the kidney and, as long as kidney function remains unimpaired, should be safe for use in normal dosages in patients with liver disease. Volume of distribution varies with total body water, which will increase in patients with ascites; as volume of distribution increases, half-life will also increase according to the relationship defined earlier [41]:

The hepatorenal syndrome is a relatively rare complication of liver disease which leads to a decline in renal function; if this should develop, lithium dosage will need to be adjusted according to the guidelines described later in this paper.

In an effort to bring a systematic approach to the problem of medication dosing in patients with liver disease, Arns et al. [10] have proposed the general guidelines presented in table 1.

Under this system drugs are described as being either flow sensitive, enzyme sensitive, or both, based on degree of first-pass extraction. Flow-limited drugs have a large intrinsic hepatic clearance relative to liver blood flow, and as such have large reserve metabolic capacities. They are sensitive to reduced delivery of drug to the metabolic sites, whether through reduced total blood to the liver or through disruptions in hepatic architecture. Enzyme-limited drugs have intrinsic hepatic clearance that is small relative to liver blood flow; the rate of extraction of these drugs is especially sensitive to the effects of disease processes that damage the metabolic activity of hepatocytes. Two additional factors are important: the extent of drug protein binding, and whether the drug is given on an acute or chronic basis. In general, enzyme-limited drugs are more sensitive to changes in the degree of protein binding than are flow-limited drugs [10].

With the exception of lithium, most psychotropics are in the enzyme-limited, binding-sensitive category of drugs, which are particularly sensitive to changes in the intrinsic metabolic functions of the impaired liver and to the effects of changes in protein binding. In addition, psychotropics are most often given on a chronic rather than acute basis. Therefore, it is reasonable to suggest that, as a general rule, when psychotropics are given to patients with liver disease, dosages should be decreased by at least 25%. In addition, serum drug levels should be carefully followed whenever possible, and close attention must be given to signs of possible drug toxicity.

In conclusion, there is general agreement that patients with severe illness are most at risk for drug-related toxicity. Cirrhosis is best studied, and cirrhotics with ascites and stigmata of liver failure sould be approached carefully when prescribing all psychopharmacologic agents. Severe acute viral hepatitis is less well studied, but caution is indicated in these patients too. With the exception of lithium, most psychotropic agents are sensitive to the effects of liver disease when it is severe. Dosages should be decreased by at least 25%, serum drug levels should be followed, and care given to signs of drug toxicity.

Psychopharmacology in Patients with Impaired Renal Function

Renal failure may be acute or more gradual in its onset. If renal failure has a rapid onset and subsequently resolves within a relatively short period of time, it is described as acute. The etiologies of acute renal failure are generally divided into prerenal (i.e. heart failure and shock), intrarenal (i.e. acute tubular necrosis), or postrenal (i.e. ureteral obstruction). Chronic renal failure has a more insidious onset with progressive and usually irreversible organ deterioration, and is most often caused by intrinsic renal disease. As renal function declines, waste products accumulate in the blood. Two of these products, blood urea nitrogen and serum creatinine, are measured as indicators of renal function, although the circulating levels of both of these products may vary with factors other than renal failure (age, muscle mass, diet, sex, etc.). Creatinine is derived from muscle catabolism and is excreted by the kidney almost unchanged. In clinical practice, creatinine clearance is generally estimated from serum creatinine by a formula correcting for the patient's age and weight:

$$\text{creatinine clearance} = \frac{(140 - \text{age})\ (\text{weight in kg})}{72 \times \text{serum creatinine (mg/dl)}}$$

Renal disease may affect the absorption, distribution, metabolism, and excretion of drugs. There are limited data available on the influence of renal disease on oral absorption of psychopharmacologic agents. Renal disease may inhibit GI absorption of drugs in several ways – for example, by higher gastric pH and impaired transport across the gastric mucosa – but the clinical significance of these effects is not well studied. However, when renal failure is secondary to decreased perfusion, as in congestive heart failure, hepatic perfusion will also be diminished and intrinsic metabolism further decreased.

Volume of distribution generally increases in renal insufficiency, largely through two mechanisms: first, total body water is usually greater in uremic patients, resulting in higher volumes of distribution for hydrophilic drugs. Secondly, serum protein binding decreases in these patients, resulting in a larger fraction of free drug, with higher volumes of distribution as well as potentially greater pharmacologic activity and toxicity. Mechanisms for this alteration in protein binding include the decrease in pH which occurs in the context of renal failure, which reduces serum protein binding through both structural and electrochemical effects. This holds true for both acidic and basic drugs, although the effect is more pronounced for acidic drugs. Additional potential mechanisms for reduced protein binding in these patients include lower total serum protein in nephrotic patients and endogenous inhibitors of protein binding [42]. For lipophilic drugs which accumulate in body fat, volume of distribution will be relatively less affected; and although uremia may decrease body fat in chronic cases, such changes do not appear to alter drug distribution significantly [43].

Drug half-life is directly related to volume of distribution and inversely related to clearance. As noted above, volume of distribution tends to increase in uremic patients, and half-life would consequently increase as a function of volume of distribution. Drug clearance, however, depends on many variables, including drug concentration, intrinsic metabolism, and excretion. Excretion is especially affected by renal disease, but may not decline as a simple ratio of decreased glomerular filtration. Most drugs are not excreted solely by glomerular filtration; many are subject to tubular secretion, which may decline at a rate different from that of glomerular filtration. Still other drugs are filtered but then reabsorbed at more distal sites, and this reabsorption also declines at an independent rate. Excretion will reflect the sum of these competing factors. For example, if reabsorption declines at a rate significantly greater than that of glomerular filtration, this would tend to maintain excretion at a rate higher than might be expected from measured glomerular filtration.

Reduced protein binding not only affects volume of distribution, as discussed above, but also affects renal elimination. Decreases in protein binding will affect glomerular filtration and tubular section differently. Bound drug does not pass through the glomerular membrane, while unbound drug is filtered freely. The concentration of unbound drug increases in uremic patients, which tends to offset the decreasing rate of glomerular filtration and maintains the rate of excretion. Tubular secretion is relatively unaffected by changes in protein binding, so that this pathway also helps maintain excretion rates in the context of failing glomerular filtration [44].

Most psychopharmacologic agents are primarily eliminated by extrarenal (especially hepatic) metabolism, so that levels of the parent drug would be expected to decline despite impaired renal function. This is especially true in the context of the decreased protein binding usually seen in uremic patients, which makes the fraction of drug available for intrinsic hepatic metabolism greater. However, the metabolites of these drugs are cleared through the kidney, and may be pharmacologically active. These active metabolites will accumulate in renal disease, and may become clinically significant. Even in the case of drugs with inactive metabolites, clinically significant effects may arise from the accumulation of these metabolites as they displace the parent drug from serum protein and compete with it for receptor sites on target tissues.

As drug elimination decreases with renal disease, modifications in drug regimens may be necessary. The safety of any drug given to a patient in renal failure will depend on a number of factors, including how much the elimination of that specific drug and of its metabolites depend on kidney function, the therapeutic index of the drug, and how readily it may be eliminated by dialysis or hemoperfusion should toxicity develop.

Clinical Considerations

Guidelines have been developed for modifying dosing regimens for patients in renal failure. In general, these guidelines are based on reductions in glomerular filtration rate as reflected by creatinine clearance. Creatinine clearance may be estimated from serum creatinine concentration, although

moderate and severe renal impairment which show no significant differences between controls and subjects with impaired renal function with respect to sertraline volume of distribution and elimination.

The monoamine oxidase inhibitors are metabolized in the liver, and have poorly characterized half-lives, volumes of distribution, and degrees of protein binding. There appears to be no need to modify dosage of MAOIs in renal failure [46], including the new reversible MAO-A inhibitor, moclobemide [51].

Anticonvulsants

In recent years carbamazepine and sodium valproate have become increasingly important in the management of patients with affective disorders. Both drugs are highly protein bound (sodium valproate 90%, carbamazepine 75%). Carbamazepine is metabolized in the liver and has active metabolites which are cleared by the kidney; sodium valproate is also metabolized in the liver, but has no known active metabolites. No adjustments in dosage are required for sodium valproate in patients with renal failure; however, carbamazepine should be decreased to 75% of normal dosage in patients with GFR less than 10 ml/min [46]. In addition to monitoring blood levels, it is advisable to follow complete blood counts (especially with carbamazepine) and liver function tests (especially with sodium valproate) when administering these drugs. Phenobarbital is eliminated by the kidney and should not be used in patients with renal failure.

Lithium

Lithium is eliminated by the kidney and may have direct nephrotoxic effects, including diabetes insipidus, renal tubular acidosis, the nephrotic syndrome, and chronic interstitial fibrosis. It may be used safely when required, but consideration should be given to other, less nephrotoxic agents when possible (see anticonvulsants, above). Levels should be followed carefully, especially as lithium has a narrow therapeutic index; as lithium is excreted unchanged, and is not protein bound, blood levels may be used very effectively as a guide to treatment. No alteration in dosage is required as long as GFR remains above 50 ml/min; when GFR is between 10 and 50 ml/min, lithium dose should be held at 50–75% of normal; and when GFR is less than 10 ml/min, dose should be 25–50% of normal [46]. In the special case of patients in complete renal failure and on dialysis, the half-life of lithium is greater than 100 h, so that these patients may be given lithium in a single dose following each dialysis treatment. The experience of Port et al. [47] suggests that pre- and postdialysis lithium levels should be monitored, and that a single lithium dose of 300–900 mg be given to the patient following treatment. They caution that a predialysis lithium level of 0.92 mEq/l should not be exceeded, as postabsorptive serum levels can be expected to be approximately 30% higher than the levels measured prior to the next dialysis.

Beta-Blockers
Atenolol and pindolol show significant accumulation in renal failure, and should be reduced to 50% of normal dose when GFR is between 10 and 50 ml/min, and to 25% of normal when GFR is less than 10 ml/min. The other beta-blockers, including propranolol, require no change in dosing regimens [46].

Calcium Channel Blockers
No modifications are required in dosages [46].

Clonidine
Clonidine dosage should be reduced to 50–75% of normal when GFR falls below 10 ml/min [46].

Psychopharmacology in Patients with Impaired Pulmonary Function

The potential adverse effects of psychopharmacologic agents on patients with pulmonary disease may be considered under two broad headings: depression of respiratory drive, and direct effects on the lung parenchyma. In general, it is the potential for depression of respiratory drive in patients with compromised pulmonary function that is more often a concern to clinicians when psychotropics are used. For the purposes of this discussion the terms 'pulmonary disease' and 'chronic obstructive pulmonary disease' (COPD) will be used interchangeably, although pulmonary disease is clearly a broader term that includes disease entities not specifically addressed here.

The exact definition of 'COPD is itself a subject of debate among specialists in pulmonary medicine [52]. We offer here the definition suggested by Snider [53], where 'COPD may be defined as a pulmonary process characterized by nonspecific changes in the lung parenchyma and bronchi, which may give rise to one or more of chronic productive cough, wheezing and dyspnea, and which may lead to emphysema and airflow obstruction.' This definition, then, includes emphysema, chronic bronchitis, and asthmatic bronchitis, as well as COPD (as more narrowly defined as a nonspecific disease of the lung parenchyma). As a measure of performance, forced expiratory volume in one second (FEV_1) is less than 1.2 liters/s [52].

Pharmacokinetic Changes in COPD

The chronic hypoxia caused by COPD has adverse physiologic effects, some of which result in altered pharmacokinetics. When CO_2 is retained serum pH declines. Most drugs are weakly ionized acids or bases, and a shift in pH alters the relative concentrations of the ionized forms of these drugs, which in turn affects drug absorption and distribution [54]. With the progression of pulmonary disease, cardiopulmonary work increases and blood flow is shifted away from splanchnic beds and the gastrointestinal tract [55]. This leads to reduced uptake of drug from the GI tract, as well as from peripheral tissue; in severe cases only drugs administered i.v. or by inhalation are reliably absorbed [54].

Drug half-life is directly dependent on volume of distribution and inversely proportional to clearance. The effects of COPD on volume of distribution and clearance of psychotropics are not well studied. The volume of distribution of theophylline compounds does not appear to change in a clinically significant way in the context of pulmonary disease [56]; however, theophylline is both less protein bound (50–60%) and has a smaller volume of distribution (0.5 liters/kg) than most psychotropics. While the clearance of theophylline appears to decrease during acute pulmonary decompensation [57], and it is reasonable to assume that this would also be the case for psychotropic medications, few data are available to support this assumption.

Clinical Considerations

Psychotropics are centrally acting drugs; in the evaluation of the adverse effects of psychotropics on patients with COPD most attention has been focused on the potential for suppression of the respiratory drive and on the potential for causing excessive sedation place period. Psychotropics are frequently used in this patient population because, as a group, patients with COPD are prone to psychiatric illness, especially depression and anxiety [58]. While some component of the etiology of these illnesses is surely situational, it is also likely that 'anxiety, restlessness, and agitation are frequently the result of hypoxia and hypoventilation caused by respiration impairment' [69]. Therefore, it is possible that attempts to alleviate a clinical situation may actually make it worse: if a tranquilizer is given to a patient to alleviate an anxiety that is at least partially caused by decreased ventilation and hypoxia, and if that tranquilizer further decreases respiratory drive, then the patient's anxiety may become more acute. This may lead to a trial of increased dose of the tranquilizer, with potentially serious consequences. Therefore, it is essential to rule out and treat hypoxia as a potential cause of anxiety before beginning psychopharmacologic treatment of a patient with COPD. In addition, as a group COPD patients tend to be older, and often suffer from a variety of additional chronic medical illnesses; all of these factors must be considered when choosing appropriate medication and making dosage decisions.

Specific Guidelines

Benzodiazepines

Of all psychotropic drugs, the benzodiazepines are probably most studied in the context of COPD. The results and recommendations derived from these studies are often contradictory, some authors finding that benzodiazepines do not appear to have adverse effects in this population of patients so long as they are used in recommended dosages [60], and others suggesting that they are dangerous drugs and should be used very cautiously, if at all [61]. These contradictory results probably reflect not so much differences among specific benzodiazepines, as differences among the patient populations studied and the method of the studies. Patients studied vary with respect to severity of pulmonary disease, age, and presence or absence of additional medical disease (especially cardiac and hepatic). Drugs studied also vary with respect to route of administration (p.o. vs. i.v.) and length of administration (acute vs. chronic).

Steen and Martinez [62] reported that 0.5-mg/kg doses of chlordiazepoxide given i.v. to healthy subjects had no significant influence on respiration; however, Model and Berry [61] found that when 10 mg t.i.d. of chlordiazepoxide was given p.o. to patients in acute respiratory failure, by the third day of treatment venous PC_{O2} was significantly increased and FEV_1 significantly decreased, and in half the sample (3 of 6 patients) the drug had to be stopped. Respiratory depression has also been found to occur after administration of diazepam to patients with COPD [63, 64]. In contrast, Kronenberg et al. [65] found no significant effect, either in terms of respiratory drive or sedation, in 6 patients with stable chronic COPD given diazepam 10 mg q.i.d. for 5 days; they speculated that diazepam was probably safe as long as it was given p.o. to patients with stable disease and without congestive heart failure.

Given the somewhat confused picture that emerges from the studies cited above, conservative managament is prudent when benzodiazepines are used to treat anxiety or agitation in patients with COPD. When benzodiazepines are indicated, they should be used for as short a time as possible, and in the lowest effective dose. Chronic use of benzodiazepines should be avoided, and they should not be used in patients with unstable pulmonary disease or hypercapnia. When stable pulmonary disease is complicated by congestive heart failure, benzodiazepines should be used with great caution. As to choice of drug, there are no studies clearly identifying the superiority of one benzodiazepine over another in this patient population. Common sense would suggest the use of drugs with shorter half-lives and fewer active metabolites, especially in patients with compromised hepatic or renal function.

Although the effects of the benzodiazepines on respiratory drive show wide individual patient-to-patient variation, the benzodiazepines are clearly more dangerous when combined with other CNS depressants [66]. Benzodiazepines should not be administered to patients with (or without) COPD who are receiving other CNS depressants, such as barbiturates or opiate analgesics, and should not be made available on a prescription basis to any patient in whom there is a likelihood of concurrent ingestion of alcohol or some other CNS depressant.

Neuroleptics

The use of neuroleptics in patients with COPD is potentially problematic. Although respiratory depression is a rare complication of the use of neuroleptics [67], when it occurs it has the potential for catastrophic results. The two main areas of concern when considering the use of neuroleptics in patients with compromised pulmonary function are sedation and acute laryngopharyngeal paresis [68, 69]; sedation is more associated with the low-potency neuroleptics, while dystonia is more frequently seen with high-potency neuroleptics.

When treating an agitated patient with COPD, it is important to identify a clear need for the use of a neuroleptic. As in the case of the benzodiazepines, it is necessary to establish whether the patient's anxiety and agitation are secondary to an underlying hypoxia, and to correct that condition first before turning to psychopharmacologic agents. For the agitated and anxious patient who is not psychotic, a short-acting benzodiazepine is probably a better choice than a neuroleptic [70]; for the severely agitated and psychotic patient, low doses of high potency neuroleptics are recommended [71]. When using any neuroleptic the possibility of an acute laryngopharyngeal dystonic reaction should be kept in mind, and all patients given (especially) high-potency neuroleptics should be covered with an anticholinergic agent, usually diphenhydramine or benztropine. When employing either anticholinergic agent, however, it should be remembered that both have antihistaminic and atropine-like activities that may thicken bronchial secretions and precipitate wheezing, especially in asthmatic patients. Consequently, it is important to adhere to the minimum possible dose of either drug.

Patients with tardive dyskinesia pose a particular problem. Tardive diskinesia may be a sequela of either low- or high-potency neuroleptics, and is usually characterized by involuntary orofacial, limb, and truncal dyskinesias, as well as respiratory grunting. However, tardive diskinesia may also be rarely associated with ventilatory compromise and sudden death [71], even in patients without primary pulmonary disease. Casey and Rabins [71] noted that in some patients, when respiratory distress was treated by decreasing neuroleptic dosages, respiratory function actually worsened. Therefore, for patients with tardive diskinesia and COPD, and who are experiencing acute respiratory distress, a withdrawal of neuroleptic may be contraindicated. For these patients a change to the new neuroleptic clozapine might be considered when the patient is clinically stable.

Antidepressants

The tricyclic antidepressants are structurally similar to the phenothiazines and, like the phenothiazines, may cause sedation. The tricyclics do not appear to depress respiratory function in healthy subjects [72]; there are very few data on their effects on patients with COPD when administered in therapeutic dosages. There are, however, extensive data on TCA overdose, and rapid progression to coma and respiratory arrest has been observed [73–76]. In addition, adult respiratory distress syndrome has occurred following tricyclic overdose [77].

Series and Cormier [78] studied the effects of protriptyline, a nonsedating tricyclic with a very long half-life, on the respiratory function of 16 patients with stable COPD and found improvement in ventilatory function and oxygenation. Bonora et al. [79] studied the activity of phrenic, hypoglossal, and recurrent laryngeal nerves in vagotomized decerebrate cats and found that protriptyline increased the activity of upper airway (hypoglossal and recurrent laryngeal) nerves, and had no effect on phrenic nerve activity; they also noted in the same study that diazepam decreased the activity of these nerves. Asthmatic patients have been observed to show clinical improvement when treated with tricyclics [80–82].

At present there are no contraindications to the use of tricyclic antidepressants in therapeutic doses in patients with stable COPD. As with the phenothiazines, sedation is the most problematic side effect in this patient population, and it would be reasonable to choose less-sedating agents such as nortriptyline, desipramine, and (especially) protriptyline.

The effects of the newer antidepressant agents, specifically bupropion and fluoxetine, are not extensively studied in this patient population. In the package insert the manufacturer of fluoxetine lists bronchitis as a 'frequent' side effect (defined as > 1/100 patients), asthma, hyperventilation and pneumonia as 'infrequent' (between 1/100 and 1/1,000 patients), and apnea and hypoxia as 'rare' events (> 1/1,000 patients). The manufacturer of bupropion describes bronchitis and dyspnea as 'infrequent' and pneumonia as 'rare'. There appear to be no case reports of patients with COPD whose symptoms were exacerbated by the use of either of these drugs.

The direct effects of these drugs on ventilatory drive in humans has not been studied. In vivo animal studies have indicated that serotonin may have central excitatory effects on inspiratory activity [83, 84].

Other Agents

The anticonvulsants (carbamazepine and valproic acid), MAOIs, and lithium do not depress respiratory function when used in therapeutic dosages. It is worth remembering, however, that elevated serum levels of many of these drugs may produce confusional states that resemble the effects of hypoxia in patients with COPD, and it is essential to follow drug levels and other applicable parameters closely.

References

1   Mendenhall CI, Robinson JD, Morgan DD: Chlordiazepoxide, librium (L), therapy in hepatic insufficiency. Gastroenterology 1975;69:845.
2   Williams RL, Mamelok RD: Hepatic disease and drug pharmacokinetics. Clin Pharmacokinet 1980;5:528–547.
3   Bircher J, Blankart R, Halpern A, Hacki W, Laissue J, Preisig R: Criteria for assessment of functional impairment in patients with cirrhosis of the liver. Eur J Clin Invest 1973;3:72–85.
4   Pirttiaho HI, Sotaniemi EA, Ahlqvist J, Pitkanen U, Pelkonen RO: Liver size and indices of drug metabolism in alcoholics. Eur J Clin Pharmacol 1978;27:465–469.
5   Desmond PV, Patwardhan RV, Johnson RF, Schenker S: Impaired elimination of caffeine in cirrhosis. Dig Dis Sci 1980;25:193–197.
6   McConnell JB, Curry SH, Davis M, Williams R: Clinical effects and metabolism of diazepam in patients with chronic liver disease. Clin Sci 1982;63:75–80.
7   Klotz U, Rapp T, Muller WA: Disposition of valproic acid in patients with liver disease. Eur J Clin Pharmacol 1978;13:55–60.
8   Benet LZ, Sheiner LB: Pharmacokinetics: the dynamics of drug absorption, distribution, and elimination; in Gilman AG, Goodman LS (eds): The Pharmacological Basis of Therapeutics. New York, MacMillan, 1985, pp 3–34.
9   Bevan JA, Thompson JH: Essentials of Pharmacology: Introduction to the Principles of Drug Action. Philadelphia, Harper & Row, 1983.
10 Arns PA, Wedlund PJ, Branch RA: Adjustment of medications in liver failure; in Chernow C (ed): The Pharmacologic Approach to the Critically Ill Patient. Baltimore, Williams & Wilkins, 1988, pp 47–68.
11 Klotz U, Fischer C, Muller-Seydlitz P, Schulz J, Muller WA: Alterations in the disposition of differently cleared drugs in patients with cirrhosis. Clin Pharmacol Ther 1979;26:221–227.
12 Shull HJ, Wilkinson GR, Johnson R, Schenker S: Normal disposition of oxazepam in acute viral hepatitis and cirrhosis. Ann Intern Med 1976;84:420–425.
13 Kraus JW, Desmond PV, Marshall JP, Johnson RF, Schenker S, Wilkinson GR: Effects of aging and liver diseases on disposition of lorazepam. Clin Pharmacol Ther 1978;24:411–419.
14 Patwardhan R, Johnson R, Sheehan J, Desmond P, Wilkinson G, Hoyumpa A, Brranch R, Schenker S: Morphine metabolism in cirrhosis. Gastroenterology 1981;80:1344.
15 Schoene B, Fleischmann RA, Remmer H: Determination of drug metabolizing enzymes in needle biopsies of human liver. Eur J Clin Pharmacol 1972;4:65–73.

16 Farrell GC, Cooksley WGE, Powell LW: Drug metabolism in liver disease: Activity of hepatic microsomal metabolizing enzymes. Clin Pharmacol Ther 1979;26:483–492.

17 Shear L, Kleinerman J, Gabuzda GJ: Renal failure in patients with cirrhosis of the liver. Am J Med 1965;39:184–198.

18 Naranjo CA, Busto U, Janecek E, Ruiz I, Roach CA, Kaplan K: An intensive drug monitoring study suggesting possible clinical irrelevance of impaired drug disposition in liver disease. Br J Clin Pharmacol 1983;15:451–458.

19 Tedesco FJ, Mills LR: Diazepam (valium) hepatitis. Dig Dis Sci 1982;27:470–472.

20 Roy-Byrne P, Vittone BJ, Uhde TW: Alprazolam-related hepatotoxicity. Lancet 1983;ii:786.

21 Seller EM, Greenblatt DJ, Giles HG, Naranjo CA, Kaplan H, MacLeod SM: Chlordiazepoxide and oxazepam disposition in cirrhosis. Clin Pharmacol Ther 1979;26:240–246.

22 Andreasen PB, Hendel J, Greisen G, Hvidberg EF: Pharmacokinetics of diazepam in disordered liver function. Eur J Clin Pharmacol 1976;10:115–120.

23 Klotz U, Antonin KH, Brugel H, Bieck PR: Disposition of diazepam and its major metabolite desmethyldiazepam in patients with liver disease. Clin Pharmacol Ther 1977;21:430–436.

24 Klotz U, Avant GR, Hoyumpa A, Schenker S, Wilkinson GR: The effects of age and liver disease on the disposition and elimination of diazepam in adult man. J Clin Invest 1975;55:347–359.

25 Ochs HR, Greenblatt DJ, Eckardt B, Harmatz JS, Shader RI: Repeated diazepam dosing in cirrhotic patients: accumulation and sedation. Clin Pharmacol Ther 1983;33:471–476.

26 Williams RL, Mamelok RD: Hepatic disease and drug pharmacokinetics. Clin Pharmacokinet 1980;5:528–547.

27 Ishak KG, Irey NS: Hepatic injury associated with the phenothiazines. Arch Pathol 1972;93:283–304.

28 Fuller CM, Yassinger S, Donlon P, Imperato TJ, Ruebner B: Haloperidol-induced liver disease. West J Med 1977;127:515–518.

29 Sherlock S: Hepatic reactions to drugs. Gut 1979;20:634–648.

30 Alexander GJ, Machiz S, Alexander RB: Phenothiazine tranquillizers: Effect of prolonged intake. Adv Exp Med Biol 1972;27:151–160.

31 Read AE, Laidlaw J, McCarthy CF: Effects of chlorpromazine in patients with hepatic disease. Br Med J 1969;iii:497–499.

32 Levinson DF, Simpson GM: Serious nonextrapyramidal adverse effects of neuroleptics: sudden death, agranulocytosis, and hepatotoxicity; in Meltzer HY (ed): Psychopharmacology: The Third Generation of Progress. New York, Raven Press, 1987, pp 1431–1436.

33 Holm E, Uhl W, Stamm S: Safety of fluvoxamine for patients with chronic liver disease: biochemical variables, psychometrics perfomance and EEG. Adv Pharmacotherapy 1986;2:151–165.

34 Golden RN, De Vane CL, Laizure SC, Rudorfer MV, Sherer MA, Potter WZ: Bupropion in depression. II. The role of metabolites in clinical outcome. Arch Gen Psychiatry 1988;45:145–149.

35 Schenker S, Bergstrom RF, Wolen RL, Lemberger LL: Fluoxetine disposition and elimination in cirrhosis. Clin Pharmacol Ther 1988;44:353–359.

36 Devane CL, Laizure SC, Stewart JT, Kolts BE, Ryerson EG, Miller RL, Lai AA: Disposition of bupropion in healthy volunteers and subjects with alcoholic liver disease. J Clin Psychopharmacol 1990;10:328–332.

37 Krastev Z, Terzilivanov D, Vlahov V: The pharmacokinetics of paroxetine in patients with liver cirrhosis. Acta Psychiatr Scand 1989;80(suppl 350):91–92.

38 Dalhoff K, Almdal TP, Bjerrum K: Pharmacokinetics of paroxetine in patients with cirrhosis. Eur J Clin Pharmacol 1991;41:351–354.

39 Stoeckel K, Pfefen JP, Mayersohn M: Absorption and disposition of moclobemide in patients with advanced age or reduced liver or kidney function. Acta Psychiatr Scand 1990;82 (suppl 360):94–97.

40 Hyman SE, Arana GW: Handbook of Psychiatric Drug Therapy. Boston, Little, Brown, 1987.

41 Brater DC, Vasko MR: Pharmacokinetics; in Chernow C (ed): The Pharmacologic Approach to the Critically Ill Patient. Baltimore, Williams & Wilkins, 1988, pp 1–20.

42 Grossman SH, Davis DD, Kitchell BB, Shand DG, Routledge PA: Diazepam and lidocaine plasma protein binding in renal disease. Clin Pharmacol Ther 1982;Mar:350–356.

43 Maher JF: Pharmacokinetic alterations with renal failure and dialysis; in Chernow C (ed): The Pharmacologic Approach to the Critically Ill Patient. Baltimore, Williams & Wilkins, 1988, pp 47–68.

44 Welling PG, Craig WA: Pharmacokinetics in disease states modifying renal function; in Benet LZ (ed): The Effect of Disease States on Drug Pharmacokinetics. Washington, American Pharmaceutical Association, 1976, pp 155–187.

45 Reidenberg MM: Renal Function and Drug Action. Philadelphia, Saunders, 1972, p 113.

46 Bennett WA, Aronoff GR, Morrison G, Golper TA, Pulliam J, Wolfson M, Singer I: Drug Prescribing in Renal Failure: Dosing Guidelines for Adults. Am J Kidney Dis 1983;3:155–183.

47 Port FK, Kroll PD, Rosenzweig J: Lithium therapy during maintenance hemodialysis. Psychosomatics 1979;20:130–131.

48 Aronoff GR, Bergstrom RF, Pottraz ST: Fluoxetine kinetics and protein binding in normal and impaired renal function. Clin Pharmacol Ther 1984;36:138–144.

49 Bergstrom RF, Beasley CM, Levey NB: Fluoxetine pharmacokinetics after daily doses of 20 mg fluoxetine in patients with severely impaired renal function. Pharm Res 1991;8(suppl 10):294.

50 Doyle GD, Laher M, Kelly JG: The pharmacokinetics of paroxetine in renal impairment. Acta Psychiatr Scand 1988;80(suppl 350):39–90.

51 Schoerlin MP, Horber FF, Frey FJ: Disposition kinetics of moclobemide, a new MAO-A inhibitor, in subjects with impaired renal function. J Clin Pharmacol 1990;30:272–284.

52 Petty TL: Definitions, clinical assessment, and risk factors; in Petty TL (ed): Chronic Obstructive Pulmonary Disease. New York, Marcel Dekker, 1985, pp 1–30.

53 Petty TL: Definitions, clinical assessment, and risk factors; in Petty TL (ed): Chronic Obstructive Pulmonary Disease. New York, Marcel Dekker, 1985, p 5.

54 Watson CB: Adjustment of Medications in Pulmonary Failure; in Chernow C (ed): The Pharmacologic Approach to the Critically Ill Patient. Baltimore, Williams & Wilkins, 1988, pp 112–130.

55 Hedley-Whyte J, Burgess GE, Feeley T: Trauma and respiratory failure; in: Applied Physiology of Respiratory Care. Boston, Little, Brown, 1976.

56 Rangno RE, Piarsky KM, Sitar D: The clinical pharmacology of theophylline and its pharmacokinetics in pulmonary edema and cirrhosis. Arzneimittelforschung 1976;26:1268–1269.

57 Vozeh S, Powell RJ, Riegelman S: Changes in theophylline clearance during acute illness. JAMA 1978;240:1882–1884.

58 Miler WF, Geumei AM: Respiratory and Pharmacological Therapy in COPD; in Petty TL (ed): Chronic Obstructive Pulmonary Disease. New York, Marcel Dekker, 1985, pp 205–338.

59 Miler WF, Geumei AM: Respiratory and Pharmacological Therapy in COPD; in Petty TL (ed): Chronic Obstructive Pulmonary Disease. New York, Marcel Dekker, 1985, pp 279.

60 Block AJ, Dolly R, Slayton PC: Does flurazepam ingestion affect breathing and oxygenation during sleep in patients with chronic obstructive lung disease? Am Rev Respir Dis 1984;129:230–233.

61 Model DG, Berry DJ: Effects of chlordiazepoxide in respiratory failure due to chronic bronchitis. Lancet 1974;ii:869.

62 Steen SN, Martinez LR: Some pharmacologic effects of intravenous chlordiazepoxide. Clin Pharmacol Ther 1964;5:44–48.

63 Catchlove RFH, Kafer ER: The effects of diazepam on respiration in patients with obstructive pulmonary disease. Anesthesiology 1971;34:14–18.

64 Clark TJH, Collins JV, Tong D: Respiratory depression caused by nitrazepam in patients with respiratory failure. Lancet 1971;ii:737–738.

65 Kronenberg RS, Cosio MG, Stevenson JE, Drage CW: The use of oral diazepam in patients with obstructive lung disease and hypercapnia. Ann Intern Med 1975;83:83–84.

66 Greenblatt DJ, Allen MD, Noel BJ, Shader RI: Acute overdosage with benzodiazepine derivatives. Clin Pharmacol Ther 1977;21:497–514.

67 Hollister LE: Adverse reactions to phenothiazines. JAMA 1964;139:143–145.

68 Flaherty JA, Lahmeyer HW: Laryngeal-pharyngeal dystonia as a possible cause of asphyxia with haloperidol treatment. Am J Psychiatry 1978;135:1414–1415.

69 Solomon K: Phenothiazine-induced bulbar palsy-like syndrome and sudden death. Am J Psychiatry 1977;134:308–311.

70 Young LD, Patl MM: Respiratory complications of antipsychotic drugs in medically ill patients. Res Staff Phys 1984;30:73–80.

71 Casey DE, Rabins P: Tardive dyskinesia as a life-threatening illness. Am J Psychiatry 1978; 135:486–488.

72 Bayliss PFC, Duncan SM: The clinical pharmacology of viloxazine hydrochloride – a new antidepressant of novel chemical structure. Br J Clin Pharmacol 1974;1:431–437.

73 Frommer DA, Kulig KW, Marx JA, Rumack B: Tricyclic antidepressant overdose. JAMA 1987;257:521–526.

74 Crome P: Antidepressant overdosage. Drugs 1982;23:431–461.

75 Nicotra MB, Rivera M, Poll JL: Tricyclic antidepressants overdose: clinical and pharmacologic observations. Clin Toxicol 1981;18:599–613.

76 Biggs JT, Spiker DG, Petit JM: Tricyclic antidepressant overdose: Incidence of symptoms. JAMA 1977;238:135–138.

77 Varnell RM, Godwin JD, Richardson ML, Vincent JM: Adult respiratory distress syndrome from overdose of tricyclic antidepressants. Radiology 1989;170:667–670.

78 Series F, Cormier Y: Effects of protriptyline on diurnal and nocturnal oxygenation in patients with chronic obstructive pulmonary disease. Ann Intern Med 1990;113:507–511.

79 Bonora M, St. John WM, Bledsoe TA: Differential elevation by protriptyline and depression by diazepam of upper airway respiratory motor activity. Am Rev Respir Dis 1985;131:41–45.

80 Ananth J: Antiasthmatic effect of amitriptyline. Can Med Assoc J 1974;110:1133.

81 Meares RA, Mills JE, Horvath TB. Amitriptyline and asthma. Med J Aust 1971;ii:25–28.

82 Wilson RCD: Antiasthmatic effect of amitriptyline. Can Med Assoc J 1974;iii:212.

83 Millhorn DE: Stimulation of raphe (obscurus) nucleus causes long term potentiation of phrenic nerve activity in cat. J Physiol 1986;381:169–179.

84 Millhorn DE, Eldridge FL, Waldrop TG: Prolonged stimulation of respiration by endogenous central serotonin. Resp Physiol 1980;42:171–188.

R. Bruce Lydiard, PhD, MD, Institute of Psychiatry, Medical University of South Carolina, 171 Ashley Avenue, Charleston, SC 29425 (USA)

Silver PA (ed): Psychotropic Drug Use in the Medically Ill.
Adv Psychosom Med. Basel, Karger, 1994, vol 21, pp 28–48

Use of Psychotropic Agents in Patients with Heart Disease

Mahlon S. Hale[a]*, Anthony Bouckoms*[b]

[a] Division of Consultation-Liaison, Psychiatry, University of Connecticut Health Center, Farmington, Conn., and
[b] Hartford Hospital, Hartford, Conn., USA

Cardiovascular disease is ubiquitous in our population and it is not uncommon for psychiatrists to be asked to assess and treat patients with concomitant psychiatric disorders and cardiovascular disease. Such interventions occur in many contexts. General hospital psychiatrists who work in coronary care units (CCUs) are familiar with patients who develop psychiatric disorders in sufficient proximity to the development or exacerbation of cardiovascular disease to support the inference of causal link, whether it be the classic cardiac neurosis, an anxiety state or a depressive condition. As with other medical conditions, it is also necessary to recognize that patients with precedent anxiety or depressive disorders are not immune from cardiovascular disorders and not surprisingly often require continued treatment of these disorders even with the complicating factor of cardiovascular ailments and their own pharmacologic treatments. The additional emergence of a large, aging population over the past decade has expanded the potential population that may be considered for treatment by psychotropic intervention. These include patients who may have suffered strokes from vascular accidents, patients who have difficulties adjusting to the regimens and restrictions of chronic disease and often patients with several, different medical disorders that require complicated pharmacologic intervention. Lastly, there is more than an interference that adequate treatment of either precedent psychiatric illness or a psychiatric component to a cardiovascular complaint will lessen morbidity and mortality [1]. The challenge for the psychiatrist who works with such patients is the selection of an intervention that promises the most benefit with the least likelihood of compromising other ongoing nonpsychiatric interventions.

In this paper, we review a number of possible pharmacologic interventions that may be used in the treatment of psychiatric disorders appearing concomitantly with or as a result of cardiovascular disease. While some patients may be suitable for psychotherapeutic treatments alone and others require joint pharmacological and verbal interventions, nonpharmacologic treatment strategies are beyond the limits of this paper. We caution that it is not possible to completely review a field such as this. For that reason, we have elected not to comment on the type A personality, as there are numerous behaviorally oriented papers that address treatment of that entity. Also, in focussing on psychopharmacologic interventions, we have had to draw some boundaries around our discussion. Anecdotal case reports of cardiac reactions to psychotropic medications abound. It is possible that by drawing the most pessimistic inference from each of these reports that all of us would be reticent to employ psychopharmacology in these patients. Such a nihilistic view is obviously as impractical as it is unwise given the morbidity that can accompany psychopathological responses to cardiovascular events. Accordingly, we have focussed on certain selected treatment issues and under each topic identified suitable agents. Thus, we address the role of classic pharmacologic interventions for depression and anxiety, the role of neuroleptics in certain syndromes, the role of newer agents, particularly in the treatment of depression, and certain notable cautions in treatment that emerged from our review of side effects and the consequences of overdoses of specific medications.

Antidepressant Drugs

In general, all antidepressants are equally efficacious for major depression. The newer monoaminergic drugs appear to have no greater efficacy than the older tricyclic and heterocyclic antidepressants, but their side effect profiles may differ. Richelson [2] has an excellent review of the receptor ligand activity of antidepressant drugs on the anticholinergic, alpha-blocking, serotonergic, norepinephrine and antihistaminic qualities of antidepressants. However, cardiac effects of antidepressants are not solely related to these receptor effects. For example, quinidine-like effects of antidepressant and neuroleptic drugs are not related to any receptor ligand activity. The effects of quinidine-like activity is to increase PR, QTc and QRS intervals.

There are some general considerations in the prescription of antidepressant medications and some specific issues for patients with cardiovascular disease. The first of these involves specific medication classes. For example, in the elderly, monamine oxidase inhibitors (MAOIs) are increasingly efficacious as tricyclics become less so. Second, atypical depression may respond better to

MAOIs then tricyclics. Third, following ECT, MAOIs seem more efficacious in preventing relapse. Yet questions of side effects and drug interactions plague the MAOIs. Clinicians need to exercise caution in their use, particularly since cardiovascular patients may be treated by many different physicians or emergently taken to hospitals when housestaff may be unfamiliar with drug usage by the patient, potential drug interactions, or even the common hypotensive side effect of these agents.

A second consideration is that certain specific diagnoses may lead to treatment algorhythms that may not be desirable for patients with heart disease. For example, panic anxiety associated with depression seems to respond best to imipramine compared to other tricyclics, but imipramine is reported to lower blood pressure twice as much as its metabolite, desipramine. Bipolar depression often presents in a mixed state with a combination of hypomania and dysphoric affect, requiring lithium in combination with an antidepressant or a neuroleptic, raising concerns about unwanted side effects.

A third consideration is that the side effect profile of a class of medications may impact directly on cardiovascular patients. We are taught that avoiding the anticholinergic, α-blocking, antihistaminic, and weight-gain-promoting effects is the key to most decisions about antidepressants. Desipramine and fluoxetine are the two best drugs in terms of minimizing anticholinergic and antihistaminic effects, while fluoxetine and nortriptyline are the least α-blocking. One should also remember that certain side effects such as sedation may have therapeutic value especially in the early stages of treatment. In recent years, there have been several extensive reviews on this subject to which the reader is referred [3].

Following some general comments below, we briefly reviewed a number of commonly used antidepressants with a specific focus on side effects relevant to the cardiovascular patient.

A partial list of antidepressants that are relatively safe for use in patients with cardiovascular disease appears in table 1.

Tricyclic Antidepressants

Early reports of doxepin's relatively safe cardiac profile led to its use in patients with cardiovascular disease [4]. These reports now appear to have been based upon studies in which low levels of medication were given (25–75 mg) [5]. The subject has been well reviewed by Jefferson [6], who came to the conclusion that the literature is not in agreement about the use of tricyclic antidepressants in patients with cardiovascular disease. It is clear that the question of tricyclic use in such patients has less to do with efficacy than with limiting the incidence of side effects, particularly those that are organ system specific.

Table 1. Selected antidepressants

Agent	Anticho-linergic effects	Sedative effects	Recommended initial daily dose mg
Doxepin	4+	4+	25
Nortriptyline	3+	2+	25
Desipramine	2+	2+	25
Trazodone	0	4+	50
Fluoxetine	0	0	10

Intensity rating: 0 = none, 4+ = high.
Adapted from Marshall and Forker [89].

In patients with cardiovascular disease, one should avoid using tricyclic antidepressants that cause either anticholinergic tachycardia or hypotension secondary to α-blockade. When initiating antidepressant therapy, do so with the appropriate safeguards in terms of prior consultations, baseline and follow-up EKGs looking for heart rate, conduction defects and the prolongation of the QTc interval. Agents that are less anticholinergic, such as the desmethylated metabolites of amitriptyline and imipramine, nortriptyline and desipramine, respectively, are advantageous. Fluoxetine competes favorably with these tricyclics in this respect since it is not anticholinergic and dosing appears to be simpler. Nonpsychiatric physicians should know that the pharmacokinetics of the two tricyclics are distinct. Nortriptyline has a 'therapeutic window' of 50–150 ng/ml [7], while desipramine response appears to mirror the linear relationship of its parent, imipramine [8]. Fluoxetine levels may vary widely between 50 and 400 ng/ml (fluoxetine + norfluoxetine), but the numbers appear to bear little relationship to efficacy or side effects.

Orthostatic Hypotension

In an important monograph, Roose and Glassman [9] reviewed the problem of hypotension caused by tricyclics. Tricyclic-induced orthostatic hypotension can be an issue in medically healthy patients and even more so in inpatients already taking hypotensive medications. In the elderly, tricyclic-induced hypotension is of further concern because there is a documented increased risk of injury from falls in older patients [10]. Orthostasis is associated with α-adrenergic blockade. In vivo findings do not always follow in vitro studies. But there are some general rules. In vivo the tertiary amines are more hypotensive than the secondary amines. Imipramine is the worst offender, while desipramine is relatively safe. The Glassman group has reported that nortriptyline and desipramine appear to lower blood pressure by about half the amount found with the tertiary amines. Clomipramine, which is currently used for obsessive-compulsive disorder has also been reported to cause noticeable hypotension. A curvilinear correlation has been found between the orthostatic drop in systolic blood pressure and plasma levels for clomipramine, but the change in orthostatic heart rate during treatment was insignificant [11].

Among tricyclics, nortriptyline and desipramine have less tendency to cause orthostatic hypotension. In a prospective study, Roose et al. [12] reported that orthostatic drop with nortriptyline averaged 14 mm Hg compared with 26 mm Hg in patients given imipramine.

Monoamine Oxidase Inhibitors

Monoamine oxidase inhibitors (MAOIs) are commonly used in psychiatry, although these drugs must be used with caution because of their high rate of drug interactions, including reactions with meperidine, tyramine-containing foodstuffs, fluoxetine and commonly used β-blockers [13]. While the most notorious side effect of MAOIs is hypertension following ingestion of foods with high tyramine content, the most common side effect of MAOIs is hypotension. Yet there is at least one report suggesting that phenelzine causes no more hypotension than nortriptyline. Georgotas et al. [14] compared 75 patients, 55 years or older, treated for major depression with either nortriptyline, phenelzine, or placebo during a 7-week period. There was a significantly greater mean orthostatic fall in systolic pressure in patients treated with nortriptyline and phenelzine as compared to the placebo group, but no significant difference was evident between the nortriptyline and phenelzine groups. The orthostatic changes appeared during the first week of treatment and were not correlated with plasma level of nortriptyline, percent platelet monoamine oxidase inhibition, or pretreatment orthostatic changes [14]. Monoamine oxidase inhibitors are apparently clear of significant cardiac side effects [15, 16]. However, given the risk of drug interactions and hypotension, MAOIs should be used cautiously in patients who are at increased risk for falls, have difficulty understanding or following dietary restrictions, or are likely to be taking other prescribed medications. To protect patients against possible drug interactions, one practical recommendation is to conduct a computerized drug interaction program for MAOIs before prescribing them in patients taking other medications. Lastly, some note must be raised about recent reports of hypertensive reactions presenting without evident causes [17].

Specific Problems with Antidepressants

Abrupt Cessation of Therapy
Caution should be exercised in the abrupt withdrawal of psychotropics in patients with cardiovascular disease. Babb et al. [18] have reported the occurrence of prolonged ventricular arrhythmias after rapid antidepressant cessation. Stevenson et al. [19] have also reported a case of ventricular fibrillation following rapid termination of lithium therapy.

Cardiac Events
Two instances of an acute myocardial infarct-like event have been described with patients taking desipramine [20, 21]. Two cases of fatal myocarditis and hepatitis associated with imipramine and its metabolite, desipramine have been reported by Morrow et al. [22]. Both cases had liver lesions associated in the medical literature with adverse drug reaction to imipramine.

Overdose Attempts and Their Consequences
Overdose concerns are an inevitable preoccupation when patients take antidepressant medications. Deaths from tricyclic antidepressant overdose are usually due to arrhythmias and/or hypotension [23]. Tricyclic toxicity is due mainly to the quinidine-like actions of these drugs on cardiac tissues. Slowing of phase 0 depolarization of the action potential results in slowing of conduction through the bundle of His and myocardium. Slowed impulse conduction is responsible for QRS prolongation and atrioventricular block, and contributes to ventricular arrhythmias and hypotension. The rough rule of thumb is that the lethal dose of most tricyclics is 2.5 g. This is one area where several of the new antidepressants offer notable advantages in terms of the potential risk, particularly in patients with preexisting cardiac disease.

Not surprisingly, the hypotensive consequences of tricyclic ingestion have been implicated in arrhythmias as well. Shannon et al. [24] reported on a group of 64 patients with tricyclic overdose. Their findings suggested thathypotension is common after severe tricyclic overdose and occurs independently of tricyclic level and prolongation of the QRS interval and that it was strongly associated with the development of arrhythmias and pulmonary edema.

Specific Medications Involved in Overdoses
The largest series of overdoses was 48 cases of fluoxetine overdose that showed that 58% had sinus tachycardia, 11% sinus bradycardia, and 21% diastolic blood pressure higher than 100 mm Hg. Incidental reports of particularly large ingestions include a report of overdose with 1,400 mg of fluoxetine that

showed a normal electrocardiogram. Another report of ingestion of 1,800 mg fluoxetine showed depressed ST segments [25].

With regard to bupropion, a further testament to its safety is that in 13 patients who overdosed (800–9,000 mg), all survived without sequelae; although the 9,000-mg patient had a seizure.

Many psychiatric patients are prescribed neuroleptic and antidepressant medications. Wilens et al. [26] reviewed their experience with 70 ICU admissions for tricyclic overdose and found that 12 had also taken a neuroleptic. This group showed a higher prevalence of first-degree atrioventricular block, a significantly higher prevalence of prolongation of the QRS duration, and a threefold increase in the prevalence of QTc prolongation. They suggested that coingestion of neuroleptics and tricyclics, when compared with the ingestion of tricyclic alone, may significantly increase the risk of adverse cardiac consequences.

With regard to the newer antidepressants, Spiller reported on 44 cases of fluoxetine and polydrug overdose showing no serious cardiac abnormalities.

Methylphenidate

Stimulant medications such as methylphenidate and dextroamphetamine have regained a role in the treatment of the elderly depressed medical patients. Cardiac effects with tachycardia and anxiety are cited as the most common reason for stopping stimulants (10%), although cardiac disease is one of the most common medical substrates on which stimulants are prescribed. Any cardiac arrhythmia represents a contraindication to stimulants. This is not so with other cardiac disease unless there is a reason to avoid the mild increase in heart rate that typically follows [27–29].

New Antidepressants

New antidepressants are often marketed on the basis of more favorable side effect profiles. Inevitably, as the use of these agents becomes widespread, case reports of various organ system side effects or side effect profiles different from the more familiar profiles of the tricyclics will appear.

New is defined as second generation, wherein the first generation are tricyclic compounds and the MAOIs. The new generation contains polycyclic, dibenzoxipine, triazolopyridine, chloropropiophenone and selective MAOIs. The particular advantages and disadvantages of each agent can be discerned by study of the neurotransmitter and receptor effects.

Fluoxetine

Fluoxetine is a new antidepressant that selectively inhibits serotonin uptake. Its major side effect is reported to be nausea reported by approximately 10–20% of patients taking fluoxetine, for which patients are advised to take the medication with meals. Twenty milligrams per day is adequate for most patients, but doses have been given in the 60 to 80-mg range. Elderly individuals may be started at 10 mg either with the elixir or by dissolving a capsule in juice and drinking half. While a few patients may require high dosages, more often simply waiting a full 6 weeks without increasing the dosage will work to optimize outcome. Fluoxetine apparently has no significant cardiac side effects [30, 31], except for rare reports of bradyarrhythmias [32, 33]. Fluoxetine does not slow intraventricular conduction, decrease blood pressure or quicken the pulse. It may slow the pulse a few beats per minute. Safety is best shown by the 663 reported cases of overdose with fluoxetine alone, in which there was only 1 death. This occurred in a woman who was estimated to have taken about 300 capsules (4,500 mg). Since fluoxetine is slowly eliminated from the body – 6 weeks is currently held as the period – extreme caution should be used when switching to an MAOI.

Cardiac Effects of Fluoxetine. Formal studies of fluoxetine's effect on the heart are limited to patients with grossly normal cardiac function, since those with unstable heart disease or recent myocardial infarction were excluded from initial studies. The only positive finding in 312 patients studied with EKGs was a mean decrease in heart rate of 3 beats/min. Significant negative findings were the absence of change in the PR and QRS intervals with fluoxetine; no conduction delays were found in any fluoxetine patients. Lastly, there are some 'spontaneous reports' that should be noted. The unknown thresholds for reporting makes this data less than of actuarial value, but it does indicate some side effects deemed worthy of report. Cardiovascular events reported more than 100 times in a population of 2,850,000 patients exposed to fluoxetine in order of greatest frequency have been hypertension, CNS hemorrhage, tachycardia, palpitations, vasodilation, syncope and hypotension. It should be noted that Spier and Frontera [33] have reported on the deaths of 3 complicated medically ill patients a short time after the institution of fluoxetine. This invokes the need for monitoring cardiac patients on fluoxetine for contraindicating its use in certain patients.

Trazodone

Trazodone is a new and chemically distinct antidepressant. It is not a tricyclic, but a trizolopyridine derivative. Trazodone is a strongly serotonergic drug in terms of S_1 and S_2 affinities and relative 5-HT uptake blockade. It has very few other significant effects except for α_1-blockade. This makes it a very good sleeping drug, yet without the anticholinergic and antihistaminic effects that often accompany sedating antidepressants. The major concern with trazodone, as with many tricyclics, is its potential for causing hypotension. It otherwise appears to be a safe agent and may offer an alternative for patients in whom conduction defects proscribe the use of tricyclics. Postural dizziness can occur but is rarely treatment limiting. Dosage is quite variable with a potential range from 50 to 600 mg/q.d. Priapism has been reported to occur in 1:6,000 cases and dissuades some from its use.

Cardiac Effects of Trazodone. When introduced, trazodone was thought to have few if any adverse cardiac effects [34]. Trazodone does not prolong the conduction time. Recently, there have been reports of increased ventricular beats in patients taking trazodone [35, 36]. Occasional case reports have appeared suggesting that ventricular tachycardia may occur [37]. Pohl et al. [38] have stated that preexisting ventricular irritability is usually present in these cases. Trazodone has also been associated with reported life-threatening premature ventricular contractions and angina in a 45-year-old white man with no prior cardiovascular disease [39].

Bupropion

This antidepressant inhibits dopamine uptake, a unique feature, and possible advantage, compared to traditional antidepressant medicines. Absence of side effects commonly experienced with tricyclics is another advantage as it is nonsedating, and is without anticholinergic effects. Lack of serotonergic uptake inhibition is a potential advantage and it has been proposed that this absence of serotonergic uptake inhibition minimizes G-I upset, anorexia, anxiety or sexual dysfunction. However, there are two properties of bupropion kinetics that complicate its use. Bupropion metabolites have long half-lives and higher plasma levels (10–100 ×) than the parent compound. This may be clinically relevant if a patient has reduced clearance due to age, altered protein binding, hepatic failure, or heart failure. Goodnick [40] showed that patients with trough levels of 10–29 ng/ml had a significantly better response than those with trough levels of 30 ng/ml or more. Blood level monitoring assumes added clinical relevance if the patient has medical reasons for impaired drug clearance such as heart failure.

Bupropion was released in 1989. This release was delayed up because of concern about a reported high incidence of seizures in some anorectic/bulimic patients. Bupropion can produce seizures, but this is uncommon (0.48% in patients treated with up to 450 mg/day for 2 years). The heightened risk is mainly in those treated with doses higher than 450 mg, where dose escalation is rapid (>100 mg/3 days), and seizure risk factors exist. Reasons for discontinuation include agitation and mental status changes 3%, G-I 2%, seizures, headache and/or sleep disturbance 2%.

Cardiac Effects of Bupropion. Currently, there is limited information about bupropion use in patients with heart disease. It has been compared favorably with amitriptyline in effect on cardiac conduction [41], and Roose et al. [42] reported on 10 depressed patients with impaired left ventricle function treated with imipramine and bupropion in a random cross-over design. Farid et al.[43] compared imipramine and bupropion and reported that hypotension requiring discontinuation of imipramine occurred in 50% of the cases; hypotension did not occurred in any of the bupropion-treated patients. More recently, Roose et al. [44] reported their findings on a 3-year study of 36 depressed patients with cardiovascular disease. In this study, buproprion was added to ongoing regimens for the treatment of preexistent illnesses. No significant conduction problems or worsening of arrhythmias were reported. But 14% of the patients did discontinue the agent because of side effects including worsening of preexistent hypertension.

There is one last caution with bupropion in patients with cardiovascular disease not because of cardiac effects *per se*, but because of its association with seizures at doses higher than those currently recommended by the manufacturer. On this basis, we would query whether bupropion should be a drug of first choice in patients at risk for seizure due to preexistent conditions.

Sertraline

Sertraline is another novel antidepressant that functions as a serotonin uptake reinhibitor. To date, sertraline is not reported to cause significant changes in pulse or in systolic or diastolic blood pressures in volunteers at therapeutic doses up to 200 mg/day. Studies of up to 400 mg have shown more side effects, especially dizziness and dry mouth.

Sertraline has been compared with amitriptyline and has a favorable cardiac safety profile with less tachycardia and hypotension than amitriptyline. Hypertension or hypotension are reported to occur in between 0.1 and 1.0% of the patients. In studies enrolling a total of 456 patients, the agent showed no demonstrable effects on intraventricular conduction or EKG time intervals.

Maprotiline

Maprotiline is a low anticholinergic agent with potent effects on blocking norepinephrine uptake. This might seem advantageous compared to some of the original tricyclics. However, maprotiline has some sedative effects from its antihistaminic profile. Clinical evidence has shown that average doses (150 mg) of maprotiline have low cardiac toxicity. Case studies showed the abeyance of premature ventricular contractions once maprotiline was started, and no worsening of conduction abnormalities in patients with preexisting conduction abnormalities [45]. Maprotiline's notoriety, however, lies in its sei-

Table 2. Selected anxiolytics

Agent	Category	Recommended initial daily dose mg
Lorazepam	benzodiazepine	1
Oxazepam	benzodiazepine	10
Alprazolam	benzodiazepine	0.25
Buspirone	azapirone	5 t.i.d.

zure-producing potential, particularly in the overdose situation. It is usually not a first-choice drug now that 'cleaner' medications are on the market. Maprotiline has been reported to cause hypotension and has been associated with heart block in patients attempting suicide by overdose [18]. These reports, coupled with numerous accounts of seizures, should exclude this drug from consideration in patients with cardiovascular disease.

Amoxapine

Amoxapine is another relatively new agent. It is related to loxapine and has been associated with extrapyramidal side effects and tardive dyskinesia in general psychiatric practice. Drug monitoring studies indicate adverse effects are mainly anticholinergic (27%) and sedative (14%). Atrial fibrillation and flutter have been reported [46, 47]. These and other risks weigh against this agent's use in patients with cardiovascular disease. In additon, this medication has a high potential for lethality, seizures, and irreversible neurological consequences when taken in overdose [48, 49].

Anxiolytics

Anxious states are commonplace in the medically ill. Table 2 contains a partial list of anxiolytic agents with relatively benign cardiac profiles. Clinicians need to consider in selection of anxiolytics whether they are treating a short-term condition, long-term trait anxiety, or one of the other anxiety conditions such as panic disorder or posttraumatic stress disorder (PTSD).

As a class, the benzodiazepines are generally safe in patients with cardiac disease [50], although caution is warranted in patients with intercurrent pulmonary conditions such as sleep apnea. Benzodiazepines have been reported to raise CO_2 levels in patients with chronic obstructive pulmonary disease. In one anecdotal report, midazolam has been implicated in sudden death as a cause of respiratory depression [51].

Major consideration regarding benzodiazepine use include their potentially extended duration of action in patients with reduced clearance or hepatic disease and the risk that their prolonged use may lead to either tolerance or sedation.

Benzodiazepines with long half-lives (2-ketobenzodiazepines) such as diazepim and chlordiazepoxide undergo oxidative metabolism. Advanced age as well as hepatic disease may complicate their metabolism and excretion. With the exception of patients with myocardial infarction, it is preferable to use shorter-acting benzodiazepines (3-hydroxybenzodiazepines). Individual preferences will distinguish use of agents such as alprazolam or lorazepam since their hepatic metabolism is less affected by concurrent illness. Psychiatrists should be aware of the need to counsel both patients and nonpsychiatric physicians regarding the wisdom of tapering these medications.

In patients with prolonged anxiety states, clinicians may wish to consider using buspirone, the azapirone derivative. The onset of this agent's action is often delayed for 2–3 weeks, and it must be taken on a regular basis (starting dose, 5 mg t.i.d.). Few drug interactions have been reported with buspirone, and it does not interact with alcohol. No EKG abnormalities have been described [52].

Neuroleptics

The use of neuroleptic drugs for the treatment of anxiety and agitation in patients with cardiovascular disease is controversial. This issue sometimes arises in patients with acute anxiety syndromes following myocardial infarcts, with delirium and with the appearance of paranoid ideation that may appear in the acute hospital setting, particularly in CCUs. Clinicians should realize that familiar low-potency neuroleptics like chlorpromazine and thioridazine are α-adrenergic blockers and can cause orthostatic hypotension. EKG changes, such as tachycardia and prolongation of the QT and PR intervals have been reported.

There are similar differences to be found in the use of neuroleptics with cardiovascular patients. Hypotension is a common phenomenon in patients taking neuroleptics [53]. Unless patients have been on these medications for prolonged periods prior to the onset of cardiovascular disease it is unwise to use either chlorpromazine or thioridazine due to the possibility of hypotension, reflex tachycardia or EKG changes mentioned above. Chlorpromazine in injectable form is thus to be absolutely avoided. One very viable alternative is the use of injectable or intravenous haloperidol (see below). Haloperidol is routinely given by some clinicians in ICUs with reportedly few complication. This topic has been reviewed by Tesar and Stern [54]. The risk of familiar short-term side effects from these medications is low. But Tesar and Stern give one noteworthy caution concerning the use of haloperidol and propanolol together from a report of subsequent hypotension and cardiopulmonary arrest [55]. Thus, while the rule should be that high-potency neuroleptics, such as perphenazine or the haloperidol, can rapidly and effectively calm highly agitated patients and can be used safely for several weeks, psychiatrists again need to be vigilant for possible drug interactions.

Haloperidol

Haloperidol is the drug of choice for delirium of uncertain etiology where symptom control of agitation or sympathetic arousal may be life threatening. As such it has a key role in the acute management of agitation in CCUs. The lack of cardiac or respiratory effect in divided i.v. doses up to 1,000 mg/day in the severely ill intensive care patient speaks for haloperidol's safety. Torsade de pointes with variable prolongation of the QRS and QT has been reported associated with haloperidol [56, 57].

New Neuroleptics

Clozapine

Clozapine has recently been reintroduced for the treatment of refractory or so-called negative symptom schizophrenia. Sedation is found in almost all patients and subjective or objective signs of orthostatic hypotension in a third [58]. These symptoms are usually mild and not treatment limiting. We suggest the low dosage of 12.5 mg be used to start treatment in patients with risk of hypotension. Sandoz Pharmaceuticals reported only 26 cases of orthostatic hypotension with syncope during the first year of use. Seizures are also reported with clozapine. This subject has been reviewed by Devinsky et al. [59] who concluded that rapid titration and high doses increased seizure risk. Dizziness and difficulty in swallowing may herald the onset of the rare, but more serious occurrence of cardiorespiratory collapse [60]. As with seizures, it appears associated with the initiation of therapy and rapid dose escalation. Again, in 12,000 cases of clozapine use, respiratory arrest or depression has been reported in 7 cases, of which only 2 involved the concomitant use of benzodiazepines. The clinical conclusion is that clozapine is usually safe, but extra care might be taken by slow initiation of therapy, avoiding benzodiazepines early in treatment, and withholding the medication if swallowing difficulty or marked nocturnal sialorrhea occurs.

Patient Groups

For the sake of this discussion, we will divide patients into those with recent myocardial infarcts and those with more chronic forms of cardiovascular diseases such as arrhythmias. Subgroups inevitably appear within these divisions and require special consideration. Geriatric patients present additional factors that must be considered in medication selection, including concurrent illnesses, metabolic changes, medication interactions, and increased medication sensitivitiy.

Patients with Myocardial Infarcts

It is very difficult to diagnose depression as opposed to a depressive reaction in the face of a major medical catastrophe such as an infarct. Although some clinicians would aggressively medicate such patients, we would withhold antidepressant medications for at least 4 weeks following the event. In the interim, the use of benzodiazepines in low doses is a reasonable means of helping patients deal with the inevitable state anxiety that accompanies these events. In this regard, the use of a familiar agent such as diazepam, which is long-acting and self-detoxifying due to its extended half-life, would be a reasonable choice. One should be wary of introducing medications that are primarily anxiolytic, but hold the promise of antidepressant activity at high doses; this outcome is questionable, and the end result may be dependency.

Treatment of the Impaired Myocardium

The question of drug selection is important in the treatment of depressed patients with impaired left-ventricular function. Roose et al. [61] compared imipramine with nortriptyline effects on ejection fraction and blood pressure in two groups (n = 21) of depressed patients with left-ventricular impairment. With both agents, the ejection fraction was unaffected, but 50% of the patients taking imipramine stopped the drug because of orthostatic hypotension, while only 1 (5%) of 21 patients taking nortriptyline dropped out. Thus, the finding of nortriptyline's relative lack of effect on blood pressure in noncardiac patients was found to extend to patients with heart disease [61].

Patients with Abnormal Cardiac Conduction

All tricyclics prolong atrial and ventricular depolarization by acting like group 1 antiarrhythmics (quinidine, procainamide) and prolonging conduction through the bundle of HIS. EKG changes may include increasing PR, QRS, QTc, and flat T waves. Initial changes in PR or QT (prolongation) do not predict ultimate changes in PR or QT and therefore risk of use. QTc changes do not increase risk until they exceed 440 ms or a 30% increase over baseline.

This subject has been extensively reviewed by Stoudemire and Atkinson [62] who present guidelines for identifying high-risk patients and for using cyclic antidepressants in patients with cardiac conduction abnormalities.

Cyclic antidepressants can produce cardiac complications in patients with certain types of cardiac conduction abnormalities. Again, most have a quinidine-like effect on the heart, which in combination with type-1 antiarrhythmic agents such as quinidine disopyramide and procainamide may induce heart block and potentially lethal arrhythmias in susceptible individuals. Patients with known cardiovascular disease warrant careful evaluation before tricyclic therapy is initiated.

Dietch and Fine [63] have also studied the cardiac effects of nortriptyline in a small sample of depressed elderly patients. Ten patients with cardiac conduction abnormalities were given therapeutic doses of nortriptyline. Serial EKGs revealed no clinically significant adverse cardiac changes. These data, added to the findings of previous research, suggest that tricyclics, in particular nortriptyline, present little risk in patients with first-degree atrioventricular block or hemiblock. Patients with bundle-branch block and bifascicular block are at greater risk of adverse cardiac sequelae but can be treated with tricyclics. To maximize safety, the authors recommend monitoring serial EKGs and plasma tricyclic levels. Ventricular irritability decreases with drugs like imipramine, so VPCs are not a contraindication. Schneider et al. [64] evaluated EKG changes with nortriptyline and 10-hydroxynortriptyline in a group of elderly depressed outpatients. They found the concentrations of nortriptyline's principal metabolite, hydroxynortriptyline, to be greater than nortriptyline in plasma. While daily nortriptyline dose and steady state plasma level in these subjects did not differ from a comparison group that did not develop conduction defects, hydroxynortriptyline levels were significantly higher. Overall, there were significant correlations between changes in the PR interval and QRS duration with plasma concentrations of nortriptyline and hydroxynortriptyline metabolites.

The general rule is that patients with isolated left bundle branch block are safe to treat with antidepressants, while much caution must be exercised in patients with second-degree block and other more complicated conditions such as atrioventricular (AV) junctional block [20].

In their review, Stoudemire and Atkinson [62] remind clinicians that cardiac consultation and an inpatient setting are the appropriate conditions for starting antidepressants in patients with complicated conduction defects. As an alternative they suggest that alternatives to antidepressants, such as alprazolam, be considered. Antidepressant activity with this medication, however, occurs at high doses and raises issues of potential dependency.

Since MAOIs are particularly useful in the elderly and the medically ill patient, it is important to remember that they do not prolong conduction time through the bundle of His. The use of MAOIs in these populations has been extensively reviewed by Robinson et al. [65–67] and Ashford and Ford [68].

A discussion of electroconvulsive therapy is beyond the scope of this chapter. Yet this form of treatment has been reported on many occasions to be safe and effective for the cardiac patient [69–71].

Arrhythmias

Although antidepressants are argued to be anti-arrhythmics, there are nonetheless multiple anecdotal reports of arrhythmias with psychotropic medications. One concern is rapid withdrawal that may occur either through inadvertence or noncompliance. Regan et al. [72] have reported arrhythmias occurring after rapid stoppage of imipramine.

Coadministration of neuroleptics and antidepressants has been anecdotally reported to cause EKG changes. This is especially true when other cardiac conduction medication is used, such as digoxin, calcium channel blockers or β-blockers. Wilens and Stern [73] have reported a case of ventricular tachycardia from desipramine and thioridazine. Importantly, they remind the reader of the effect of neuroleptics upon antidepressant plasma levels that may predispose patients to conduction difficulties [74, 75].

One of the more concerning arrhythmias is torsade de pointes. Torsade de pointes is characterized by polymorphous electrocardiographic appearance and delayed repolarization (prolonged QT interval). Psychotropics that have been implicated include haloperidol [76], thioridazine [77], and trifluoperazine [78]. It may occur in association with a number of disease states and also as a complication of treatment with therapeutic doses of drugs that affect repolarization (quinidine, disopyramide, procainamide, and phenothiazines). Clinical outcomes range from asymptomatic, self-terminating arrhythmias to ventricular fibrillation resulting in cardiac arrest. The definitive emergency therapy for torsade de pointes is overdrive pacing; cautious isoproterenol administration can also be used. Lidocaine and bretylium are often ineffective in treating this form of ventricular tachycardia. Potassium and magnesium repletion appear to be essential in abolishing drug-induced torsade de pointes. Drug-induced torsade de pointes is best prevented by avoiding agents known to induce arrhythmias in patients with a pre-existing prolonged QT interval [79]. Periodic serum electrolyte assessment (including Mg^{2+} and Ca^{2+}) is warranted, and new drugs that prolong the QTc interval should be considered potential causative agents of torsade de pointes. While other treatments such as atrial pacing are outside the scope of this chapter [80], readers should be cautioned to ask for reevaluation of EKG in patients with pre-existing prolonged QT intervals.

When all has been said, the risk that a patient may develop an arrhythmia does not necessarily rule out the use of antidepressant medications. To repeat, clinical studies and case reports have shown that nortriptyline and imipramine exert type-1 antiarrhythmic properties when plasma concentrations are therapeutic, indicating that clinical reservation against their use in cardiac patients may be overstated. A single case report by Colenda [81] describes the use of amitriptyline in a patient with arrhythmias and affective disorder without event. A general review is given by Manoach et al. [82].

Geriatric Patients

Elderly patients probably consume more prescribed drugs than does any other age-defined population symptom relief, particularly of pain, with over-the-counter medications [83]. The elderly also use large numbers of over-the-counter medications, whose side effects may complicate the use of psychotropics. The general problems entailed in prescribing psychotropic drugs for the elderly was reviewed by Thompson et al. [84] and Rockwell et al. [85] have addressed specific issues with antidepressant usage in that population. The possibility of drug interactions from known and unknown agents is thus very real. Vestal has pointed out that older patients often seek symptom relief, particularly of pain, with over-the-counter medications [86]. Unhappily, even a persevering line of questions may not elicit every medication a patient is taking from an elderly patient.

With regard to acute, inpatient conditions, it is almost axiomatic that elderly patients are more likely to be delirious in hospital than are younger patients. This high rate of delirium in the elderly may be either a result of intercurrent illness, drug reactions, brain vulnerability or stress. A good general rule to follow with elderly patients is to be cautious in the initiation of anticholinergic, sedative and α-blocking medications, particularly where the sensorium is clouded. We mention elsewhere the utility of low-dose haloperidol for anxiety and agitation. Starting treatment at low doses (1 mg b.i.d.) reduces the possibility of adverse reactions and allows clinicians to gauge the patient's tolerance for these medications.

Stroke

Antidepressant Treatment – Poststroke Depression. Depression is a serious common complication of stroke. Tricyclics as well as other antidepressants have a significant role to play [87]. Robinson's group have published extensively in this area [88]. They reported that patients with depression who are not treated with antidepressant medication did more poorly in physical and cognitive rehabilitation than patients treated with antidepressant medications. Both nortriptyline and trazodone have been reported to be efficacious.

Drug Interactions

Polypharmacy is frequently the rule in cardiovasular patients. Consequently, the use of other medications that might have similar physiologic effects or interactions with the antidepressants should always be kept in mind. Three particular situations to remember are: First, do not use MAOIs with meperidine. Second, be careful about a possible synergistic interaction between antidepressants and drugs that slow cardiac conduction or lower blood pressure. For example, some cardiac drugs like clonidine or the β-blockers may decrease the efficacy of antidepressants. Third, do not institute MAOIs with fluoxetine for 6 weeks after stopping fluoxetine. Fourth, avoid clonidine, α-methyl dopa and where possible avoid β-blockers in patients taking antidepressants. Fifth, remember that carbamazepine will tend to decrease the levels of other medications including antidepressants.

Selection of appropriate antidepressant or anxiolytic medications is more complex in patients with cardiovascular disease than in patients without medical illnesses. The need for cautious review of underlying physiologic issues, potential drug interactions, and concerns about specific side effects, however, is as critical in patients with cardiovascular disease as in those with illnesses involving other organ systems. Rational treatment decisions should be made that take into account both the pathophysiology of the underlying cardiovascular illness and the potential benefits that result from improving mood and relieving anxiety. Experience has shown that alleviation of depression and anxiety greatly improves patient welfare and outcome. Failure to treat depression and anxiety multiplies morbidity and mortality from cardiovascular disease.

References

1   Weeke A, Juel K, Vaeth M: Cardiovascular death and manic-depressive psychosis. J Affective Disord 1987; 13:287–292.
2   Richelson E: Antidepressants and brain neurochemistry. Mayo Clin Proc 1990;64:1227–1236.
3   Roose SP, Glassman AH, Dalack GW: Depression, heart disease, and tricyclic antidepressants. J Clin Psychiatry 1989;50(suppl):12–16.
4   Burrows GD, Vohra J, Dumovic P, et al: TCA drugs and cardiac conduction. Prog Neuropsychopharmacol 1977;1:329–334.
5   Luchins DJ: Review of clinical and animal studies comparing the cardiovascular effects of doxepin and other tricyclic antidepressants. Am J Psychiatry 1983;140:1006–1009.
6   Jefferson JW: Cardiovascular effects and toxicity of anxiolytics and antidepressants. J Clin Psychiatry 1989;50:368–378.
7   Asberg M, Cronholm B, Sjoqvist F, et al: Relationship between plasma level and therapeutic effect of nortriptyline. Br Med J 1971;iii:331–334.
8   Nelson JC, Jatlow P, Quinlan DM, et al: Desipramine plasma concentration and antidepressant response. Arch Gen Psychiatry 1982;39:1419–1422.
9   Roose SP, Glassman AH: Cardiovascular effects of tricyclic antidepressants in depressed patients with and without heart disease. J Clin Psychiatry Monograph 1989;7:1–18.

10   Ray WA, Griffin MR, Schafner W, et al: Psychotropic drug use and the risk of hip fracture. N Engl J Med 1987;316:363–369.

11   Christensen P, Thomsen HY, Pedersen OL, Gram LF, Kragh-Srensen P: Orthostatic side effects of clomipramine and citalopram during treatment for depression. Psychopharmacology (Berl) 1985;86:383–385.

12   Roose SP, Glassman AH, Siris SG, et al: Comparison of imipramine and nortriptyline induced orthostatic hypotension: A meaningful difference. J Clin Psychopharmacol 1981;1:316–319.

13   Reggev A, Vollhardtn BR: Bradycardia induced by an interaction between phenelzine and beta blockers. Psychosomatics 1989;30:106–108.

14   Georgotas A, McCue RE, Friedman E, Cooper TB: A placebo-controlled comparison of the effect of nortriptyline and phenelzine on orthostatic hypotension in elderly depressed patients. J Clin Psychopharmacol 1987;7:413–416.

15   McGrath PJ, Blood DK, Stewart JW, et al: A comparative study of the electrocardiographic effects of phenelzine, tricyclic antidepressants, mianserin, and placebo. J Clin Psychopharmacol 1987;7:335–339.

16   Goldman LS, Alexander RC, Luchins DJ: Monoamine oxidase inhibitors and tricyclic antidepressants: Comparison of their cardiovascular effects. J Clin Psychiatry 1986;47:225–229.

17   Fallon B, Foote B, Walsh BT, Roose SP: 'Spontaneous' hypertensive episodes with monoamine oxidase inhibitors. J Clin Psychiatry 1988;49:163–165.

18   Babb SV, Dunlop SR, Hoffmann MA: Protracted ventricular arrhythmias occurring after abrupt tricyclic antidepressant withdrawal. Psychosomatics 1990;31:452–454.

19   Stevenson RN, Blanshard C, Patterson DL: Ventricular fibrillation due to lithium withdrawal: An interaction with chlorpromazine? Postgrad Med J 1989;65:936–938.

20   Borganelli M, Forman MB: Simulation of acute myocardial infarction by desipramine hydrochloride. Am Heart J 1990;119:1413–1414.

21   Smith DB, Tyznik JW: Desipramine-induced conduction disorder mimicking myocardial infarction. Postgrad Med 1987;82:86–88.

22   Morrow PL, Hardin NJ, Bonadies J: Hypersensitivity myocarditis and hepatitis associated with imipramine and its metabolite, desipramine. J Forensic Sci 1989;34:1016–1020.

23   Pellinen TJ, Farkkila M, Heikkila J, Luomanmaki K: Electrocardiographic and clinical features of tricyclic antidepressant intoxication. A survey of 88 cases and outlines of therapy. Ann Clin Res 1987;19:12–17.

24   Shannon M, Merola J, Lovejoy FH Jr: Hypotension in severe tricyclic antidepressant overdose. Am J Emerg Med 1988;6:439–442.

25   Riddle MA, Brown N, Dzubinski D, Jetmalani AN, et al: Fluoxetine overdose in an adolescent. J Am Acad Child Adolesc Psychiatry 1989;28:587–588.

26   Wilens TE, Stern TA, Ogara PT: Adverse cardiac effects of combined neuroleptic ingestion and tricyclic antidepressant overdose. J Clin Psychopharmacol 1990;10:51–54.

27   Chiarello RJ, Cole JO: The use of psychostimulants in general psychiatry. Arch Gen Psychiatry 1987;44:286–295.

28   Masand P, Pickett P, Murray GB: Psychostimulants for secondary depression in medical illness. Psychosomatics 1991;32:203–208.

29   Pickett P, Masand P, Murray GB: Psychostimulant treatment of geriatric depressive disorders secondary to medical illness. J Neurol 1990;3:146–151.

30   Cooper GL: The safety of fluoxetine: An update. Br J Psychiatry 1988;153(3, suppl):77–86.

31   Fish C: Effect of fluoxetine on the electrocardiogram. J Clin Psychiatry 1985;46:42–44.

32   Buff DD, Brenner R, Kirtane SS, Gilboa R: Dysrhythmia associated with fluoxetine treatment in an elderly patient with cardia disease. J Clin Psychiatry 1991;52:174–176.

33   Spier SA, Frontera MA: Unexpected deaths in depressed medicalinpatients treated with fluoxetine. J Clin Psychiatry 1991;52:377–382.

34   Himmelhoch JM, Schechtman K, Auchenbach R: The role of trazodone in the treatment of depressed cardiac patients. Psychopathology 1984;17(2, suppl):51–63.

35   Janowsky D, Curtis G, Zisook S, et al: Ventricular arrhythmias possibly aggravated by trazodone. Am J Psychiatry 1983;140:796–797.

36   Aronson MD, Hafex H: A case of trazodone-induced ventricular tachycardia. J Clin Psychiatry 1986;47:388–389.

37   Vitullo RN, Wharton JM, Allen NB, Pritchett EL: Trazodone related exercise induced nonsustained ventricular tachycardia. Chest 1990;98:247–248.

38   Pohl R, Bridges M, Rainey JM, et al: Effects of trazodone and desipramine on cardiac rate and rhythm in a patient with preexisting cardiovascular disease. J Clin Psychopharmacol 1986;6: 380–381.

39   Aronson MD, Hafez H: A case of trazodone-induced ventricular tachycardia. J Clin Psychiatry 1986;47:388–389.

40   Goodnick PJ: Blood levels and acute response to bupropion. Am J Psychiatry 1992;149:399–400.

41   Wenger TL, Cohn JB, Bustrack J: Comparison of the effects of bupropion and amitriptyline on cardiac conduction in depressed patients. J Clin Psychiatry 1983;44:174–175.

42   Roose SP, Glassman AH, Giardina EG, Johnson LL, Walsh BT, Bigger JT Jr: Cardiovascular effects of imipramine and bupropion in depressed patients with congestive heart failure. J Clin Psychopharmacol 1987;7:247–251.

43   Farid F, Wenger T, Siingh B, Ely E: Use of bupropion in patients who exhibit orthostatic hypotension on tricyclic antidepressants. J Clin Psychiatry 1983;44:170–173.

44   Roose SP, Dalack GW, Glassman AH, Woodring S, Walsh T, Biardina EGV: Cardiovascular effects of bupropion in depressed patients with heart disease. Am J Psychiatry 1991;148:512–516.

45   Ghadirian AM, Ananth J: Safety of maprotiline in treatment of cardiac patients with left anterior hemiblock. Psychiatr J Univ Ott 1989;14:476–477.

46   Zavodnick S: Atrial flutter with amoxapine: A case report. Am J Psychiatry 1981;138: 1503–1505.

47   Murray AB: Atril fibrillation/flutter associated with amoxapine: Two case reports. J Clin Psychopharmacol 1985;198:124–125.

48   Litovitz JL, Troutman WG: Amoxapine overdose: A case report. Am J Psychiatry 1982;139:1619–1620.

49   Bock JL, Cummings KC, Jatlow PI: Amoxapine overdose: A case report. Am J Psychiatry 1982; 139:1619–1620.

50   Stern TA, Caplan RA, Cassem NH: Use of benzodiazepines in a coronary care unit. Psychosomatics 1987;28:19–23.

51   Taylor JW, Simon KB: Possible intramuscular midazolam associated cardiorespiratory arrest and death. DICP 1990;24:695–697.

52   Murasaki M, Miura S, Ishigooka J, Ishii Y, Takahashi A, Fukuyama Y: Phase I study of a new antianxiety drug, buspirone. Prog Neuropsychopharm Biol Psychiatry 1989;13:137–144.

53   Silver H, Kogan H, Zlotogorski D: Postural hypotension in chronically medicated schizophrenics. J Clin Psychiatry 1990;51:459–462.

54   Tesar GE, Stern TA: Rapid tranquilization of the agitated intensive care patient. J Intens Care Med 1988;3:195–201.

55   Alexander HE, McCarty K, Giffen MB: Hypotension and cardiopulmonary arrest associated with concurrent haloperidol and propranolol therapy. JAMA 1984;252:87–88.

56   Fayer SA: Torsades de pointes ventricular tachyarrhythmia associated with haloperidol. J Clin Psychopharmacol 1986;6:375–376.

57   Kriwisky M, Perry GY, Tarchitsky D, Gutman Y, Kishon Y: Haloperidol-induced torsades de pointes. Chest 1990;98:482.

58   Baldessarini RJ, Frankenburg FR: Clozapine: A novel antipsychotic agent. N Engl J Med 1991; 324:746–754.

59   Devinsky O, Honigfeld G, Patin J: Clozapine-related seizures. Neurology 1991;41:369–371.

60   Friedman LJ, Tabb SE, Worthington JJ, Sanchez CJ, Sved M: Clozapine: A novel antipsychotic agent (letter, comment). N Engl J Med 1991;325:518–519.

61   Roose SP, Glassman AH, Giardina EG, Johnson LL, Walsh EBT, Woodring S, Bigger JT Jr: Nortriptyline in depressed patients with left ventricular impairment. JAMA 1986;256: 3253–3257.

62   Stoudemire A, Atkinson P: Use of cyclic antidepressants in patients with cardiac conduction disturbances. Gen Hosp Psychiatry 1988;10:389–397.

63   Dietch JT, Fine M: The effect of nortriptyline in elderly patients with cardiac conduction disease. J Clin Psychiatry 1990;51:65–67.

64 Schneider LS, Cooper TB, Severson JA, Zemplenyi T, Sloane RB: Electrocardiographic changes with nortriptyline and 10-hydroxynortriptyline in elderly depressed outpatients. J Clin Psychopharmacol 1988;8:402–408.
65 Robinson DS: Age-related factors affecting antidepressant drug metabolism and clinical response; in Nandy K (ed): Geriatric Psychopharmacology. New York, Elsevier/North-Holland, 1979.
66 Robinson DS, Nies A, Coretta J, Cooper TB, Spencer C: Cardiovascular effects of phenelzine and amitriptyline in depressed outpatients. J Clin Psychiatry 1982;43:8–15.
67 Robinson DS, Sourkes JL, Nies A: Monoamine metabolism in human brain. Arch Gen Psychiatry 1977;34:89–92.
68 Ashford JW, Ford CV: Use of MAO inhibitors in elderly patients. Am J Psychiatry 1979;136: 1466–1467.
69 Drop JD, Welch CA: Anesthesia for electroconvulsive therapy in patients with major cardiovascular risk factors. Convuls Ther 1989;5:88–101.
70 Drop LJ, Bouckoms AJ, Welch CA: Arterial hypertension and multiple cerebral aneurysms in a patient treated with electroconvulsive therapy. J Clin Psychiatry 1988;49:280–282.
71 Alexopoulos GS, Frances RJ: ECT and cardiac patients with pacemakers. Am J Psychiatry 1980;137:1111–1112.
72 Regan WM, Margolin RA, Mathew RJ: Cardiac arrhythmia following rapid imipramine withdrawal. Biol Psychiatry 1989;25:482–484.
73 Wilens E, Stern TA: Ventricular tachycardia associated with desipramine and thioridazine. Psychosomatics 1990;31:100–103.
74 Nelson JC, Jatlow PF: Neuroleptic effect on desipramine steady state plasma concentrations. Am J Psychiatry 1980;137:1232–1234.
75 Hirschowitz J, Bennett JA, Zemlan FP, et al: Thioridazine effect on desipramine plasma levels. J Clin Psychopharmacol 1983;3:376–379.
76 Kriwisky M, Perry GY, Tarchitsky D, et al: Haloperidol-induced torsades de pointes. Chest 1990;98:482–484.
77 Kiriike N, Maeda Y, Nishiwaki S, Izumiya Y, Katahara S, Mui K, Kawakita Y, Nishikimi T, Takeuchi K, Takeda T: Iatrogenic torsade de pointes induced by thioridazine. Biol Psychiatry 1987;22:99–103.
78 Raehl CL, Patel AK, LeRoy M: Drug-induced torsade de pointes. Clin Pharmacol 1985;4:675–690.
79 Flugelman MY, Tal A, Pollack S, et al: Psychotropic drugs and long QT syndromes: case reports. J Clin Psychiatry 1985;46:290–291.
80 Davison ET: Amitriptyline induced torsade de pointes: Successful therapy with atrial pacing. J Electrocardiol 1985;18:299–301.
81 Colenda CC: Antiarrhythmic properties of amitriptyline. South Med J 1990;83:78–80.
82 Manoach M, Varon D, Neuman M, Erez M: The cardioprotective features of tricyclic antidepressants. Gen Pharmacol 1989;20:269–275.
83 Vestal RE: Drug use in the elderly: A review of problems and special considerations. Drugs 1978;16:358–382.
84 Thompson TL, Moran MG, Nies AS: Psychotropic drug use in the elderly. N Engl J Med 1983; 308:194–199.
85 Rockwell E, Lam RW, Zisook S: Antidepressant drug studies in the elderly. Psychiatr Clin North Am 1988;11:215–233.
86 Chien CP, Townsend EJ, Ross-Townsend A: Substance use and abuse among the community elderly: The medical aspect. Addict Dis 1978;3:357–372.
87 Catapano F, Galderisi S: Depression and cerebral stroke. J Clin Psychiatry 1990;51(9, suppl):9–12.
88 Fedoroff JP, Robinson RG: Tricyclic antidepressants in the treatment of poststroke depression. J Clin Psychiatry 1989;50(suppl):18–23.
89 Marshall JB, Forker AD: Cardiovascular effects of tricyclic antidepressant drugs: Therapeutic usage, overdose, and management of complications. Am Heart J 1982;103:401–414.

Mahlon S. Hale, MD, Divison of Consultation-Liaison Psychiatry,
University of Connecticut Health Center, Farmington, CT 06030 (USA)

Silver PA (ed): Psychotropic Drug Use in the Medically Ill.
Adv Psychosom Med. Basel, Karger, 1994, vol 21, pp 49–60

Psychotropic Medications in Gastrointestinal and Hepatic Disease

Steven A. Epstein

Department of Psychiatry, Georgetown University Medical Center,
Washington, D. C., USA

Gastrointestinal symptoms are among the most common reasons for seeking care from general medical practitioners. A number of gastrointestinal diseases, such as irritable bowel syndrome and esophageal motility disorders, have a significant degree of psychiatric comorbidity. When using pharmacotherapy for any patients with gastrointestinal disease, one must be aware of the gastrointestinal side effects of these medications as well as drug interactions with medications used to treat the primary medical disorders. Psychotropic medications may also be used to treat gastrointestinal problems, e.g. tricyclic antidepressants for irritable bowel syndrome. Because psychotropic medications are virtually always given by mouth and metabolized by the liver, diseases of this system may affect absorption and metabolism. This chapter will address these issues as they pertain to the major gastrointestinal organ systems. It concludes with a brief discussion of parenteral pharmacotherapy in patients who cannot take medications orally.

Esophageal Disorders

Mood disorders and generalized anxiety disorder are often seen in persons with esophageal motility disorders [1, 2]. Globus, the sensation of a lump in one's throat, may be associated with panic disorder and depression [3]. It is not surprising that psychopharmacologic treatment of anxiety or depression often helps these patients by reducing their psychiatric symptomatology. In addition, esophageal symptoms may be diminished by pharmacotherapy. For example, the globus sensation has been shown to be responsive to antidepressants [4], and trazodone has been found to be helpful in the esophageal spasm syndrome [5, 6].

Hiatal hernia and resultant gastroesophageal reflux are commonly seen in the general medical setting. In one study, patients with gastroesophageal reflux appeared to be more depressed than a comparison group with similar symptoms but without physical evidence of reflux [7]. Any medication with anticholinergic effects may exacerbate gastroesophageal reflux. Thus, for treatment of depression in this population one should use tricyclics with the least anticholinergic effects or consider agents without anticholinergic effects (e.g. fluoxetine, bupropion, MAO inhibitors). High potency neuroleptics would be preferred in the treatment of psychosis.

Gastric Disorders

There is generally little to be concerned about when using psychotropic medications in patients with peptic ulcer disease and gastritis. The tricyclic antidepressants doxepin and trimipramine, both potent H-2 blockers, have been found to be helpful in peptic ulcer disease [8, 9]. (Though their mechanism of action probably includes H-2 receptor inhibition, this has not been fully elucidated [10].) Thus, in a patient with ulcer disease and depression, a tricyclic agent such as doxepin would be an excellent choice.

Gastroparesis may be a problem for persons with such conditions as diabetes mellitus and pyloric stenosis. Highly anticholinergic psychotropic agents (e.g. benztropine, low-potency neuroleptics, and tertiary amine tricyclic antidepressants) theoretically could cause or exacerbate this condition, especially in high-risk patients [11]. Thus, with these patients it is prudent to avoid psychotropic drugs with significant anticholinergic effects. If an antidepressant must be used, one could use a minimally anticholinergic tricyclic such as nortriptyline, or nontricyclics such as fluoxetine, bupropion, or a monoamine oxidase inhibitor. A high potency neuroleptic such as haloperidol or fluphenazine would be preferred for psychosis.

Drug interactions involving gastric medications and psychotropic medications may be quite significant. Antacids have been shown to decrease the rate of absorption of chlordiazepoxide [12] and diazepam [13] in single-dose studies. Thus, peak clinical effects may be diminished when a single dose of these medications is taken with an antacid. However, chronic use of clorazepate and an antacid has been shown not to affect steady state levels [14]. The mechanism of decreased absorption likely lies in decreased gastric emptying due to the antacid [15]. Chlorpromazine absorption is impaired by the co-administration of an antacid [16], but interactions with other antipsychotics have not been clearly established.

Cimetidine, an H-2 antagonist widely used to treat peptic ulcer disease, interacts significantly with a number of psychotropic agents because it inhibits oxidative hepatic metabolism. It has been shown to increase the blood level of imipramine [17]. Diazepam levels [18] and chlordiazepoxide levels [19] have also been shown to be increased by cimetidine. If benzodiazepines need to be used with cimetidine, it is prudent to use one that is metabolized by conjugation (lorazepam, oxazepam, or temazepam) [15]. Transient increases in carbamazepine levels can occur when one adds cimetidine [20].

Other H-2 blocking agents have fewer psychotropic drug interactions than cimetidine. Ranitidine does not impair the clearance of lorazepam, diazepam [21] or carbamazepine [22]. Famotidine and nizatidine are two new H-2 antagonists which appear to be efficacious in the treatment of ulcer disease [23, 24]. Famotidine does not affect the hepatic mixed-function oxidase systems [25]. Though nizatidine interactions have not been elucidated, there is no evidence to suggest that they will be different from those of ranitidine [24]. The new drug omeprazole is approved in the United States for extended use in pathologic hypersecretory states such as Zollinger-Ellison syndrome and for refractory gastroesophageal reflux. Omeprazole inhibits the oxidative metabolism of drugs such as diazepam [26].

Many psychotropic medications have the potential to cause nausea and/or vomiting. Mood-stabilizing agents are often associated with this side effect. Lithium may cause nausea and vomiting at therapeutic levels. However, these effects occur more commonly when dosages are rapidly increased [27]. They may be minimized by gradual dose increases, taking lithium with food, and lowering serum levels if clinically appropriate. Lithium citrate and longer acting forms such as Lithobid appear to cause fewer gastric side effects than does lithium carbonate. Carbamazepine may cause nausea, particularly at peak levels which occur 2–3 h after a dose. Dividing dosages may help minimize this side effect [28]. Sodium valproate may occasionally cause gastrointestinal complaints such as abdominal cramps [29]. Converting to Depakote (divalproex sodium), which is enteric-coated, may help minimize the occurrence of this side effect [30].

Fluoxetine causes nausea in up to 25% of patients but rarely leads to vomiting [31]. However, tolerance may often develop in 1–2 weeks [32]. In a retrospective report, clomipramine caused nausea in 39% of patients with obsessive-compulsive disorder [33]. However, in a recent controlled study in persons with obsessive-compulsive disorder nausea was not a major side effect with either clomipramine or fluoxetine [34]. Discontinuation of antipsychotics and tricyclic antidepressants may lead to gastrointestinal distress but this can be minimized by slowly tapering these agents [27].

Small Intestine and Colon

The small intestine is the site of absorption of most psychotropic drugs. Therefore, at least in theory, diseases primarily affecting the small intestine, such as celiac disease, could affect the absorption of psychotropic drugs. One study showed that lithium absorption occurs entirely in the small intestine [35]. Therefore, lithium absorption could decrease when intestinal transit time decreases as in diarrhea [11]. However, there are no other specific studies regarding absorption of other psychotropic agents. If there is a suspicion of malabsorption, one could monitor blood levels of the particular agent [11].

Irritable bowel syndrome and inflammatory bowel disease are the main intestinal diseases of interest to psychiatrists. There are generally no limitations to the use of psychoactive medications in these conditions. However, one would be prudent to avoid medications with significant anticholinergic effects in the constipation-predominant form of irritable bowel syndrome and when a person with ulcerative colitis is at risk for toxic megacolon. In addition, it is unwise to give lithium to persons with ulcerative colitis because of its tendency to increase diarrhea.

Irritable bowel syndrome may be due to abnormal myoelectrical activity of the colon [36]. However, there is a good deal of evidence that psychiatric factors play a role in the illness. Persons with irritable bowel syndrome have been found to be more depressed and anxious than normal controls. In addition, one study has found that 28% of patients met criteria for somatization disorder [37]. Psychiatric illness often precedes gastrointestinal symptoms, suggesting that psychological comorbidity is not merely a reaction to illness [38]. It is interesting to note, however, that non-patients who meet diagnostic criteria for irritable bowel syndrome do not have increased psychiatric problems [39]. Therefore, persons with such symptoms may seek medical care because of the presence of some degree of abnormal illness behavior.

Treatments for irritable bowel syndrome include high-fiber diet, bulking agents, anticholinergic agents (for the diarrhea-predominant form), tricyclic antidepressants, minor tranquilizers, psychotherapy and education [40]. Because pharmacotherapy studies have been so poorly designed, it is difficult to state the efficacy of any particular psychotropic agent [41]. Clinical experience indicates that antidepressants are often helpful even when the patient is not depressed. For diarrhea-predominant irritable bowel syndrome, highly anticholinergic antidepressants are preferred; for the constipation-predominant form, an agent with low or no anticholinergic effects is recommended. Anxiolytics are often helpful when there is concomitant anxiety. There is a significant comorbidity of irritable bowel syndrome and panic disorder. In patients with both disorders, gastrointestinal symptoms respond to antipanic medications [42, 43].

One of the frequent mainstays of treatment of irritable bowel syndrome is the use of an antispasmodic agent. It is important for the psychiatrist to be aware of the constituents of such agents, since they include substances of potential interest. For example, one must use caution in prescribing a medication with significant anticholinergic effects when a patient is taking any of a number of antispasmodic agents. Bentyl (dicyclomine) and Probanthine (propantheline) are anticholinergic agents. Levsin (hyoscyamine) has anticholinergic effects as well. Donnatal includes phenobarbital (16 mg), atropine, scopolamine, and hyoscyamine. Librax includes chlordiazepoxide and the anticholinergic/spasmolytic clinidium. Though one tablet of Librax contains only 5 mg of chlordiazepoxide, the psychiatrist must be cautious in prescribing other sedative/hypnotics, particularly in the elderly. Phenobarbital can affect blood levels of psychotropic agents and of course can be quite sedating.

The antidiarrheal agent Lomotil contains atropine and diphenoxylate, which is chemically related to meperidine. Thus one must be aware that a patient taking this medication is receiving an anticholinergic agent and an opiate. Since diphenoxylate is structurally similar to meperidine there is a theoretical potential for precipitation of a hypertensive crisis with the concomitant use of an MAO inhibitor. However, no cases of such an interaction have been reported.

Ulcerative colitis (UC) was once considered to be a psychosomatic disease. However, a recent review found methodologic flaws in virtually all studies examining associations between UC and psychiatric factors [44]. None of the well-controlled studies [e. g., 45] found an association. It does appear, however, that there is greater psychiatric comorbidity in Crohn disease than UC. For example, a recent study using the Diagnostic Interview Schedule found that Crohn disease patients but not UC patients had a greater prevalence of anxiety and depression than controls [45]. When steroids are used for either condition, the patient must be monitored for an organic mood disorder, particularly if there is a premorbid history of a mood disorder or of mood changes with prior steroid therapy.

Constipation and diarrhea are the main colonic side effects of psychotropic agents. Tricyclic antidepressants, trazodone, bupropion and monoamine oxidase inhibitors are prone to cause constipation. There are a number of alternatives to consider if constipation becomes a serious problem. Secondary amine tricyclics such as nortriptyline and desipramine are less likely to cause constipation than tertiary amines. Fluoxetine appears to cause constipation infrequently. Antipsychotics may cause constipation, though usually to a lesser extent than tricyclic antidepressants because of their overall lower anticholinergic activity. Higher potency neuroleptics are preferred. The anticholinergic agents benztropine and trihexyphenidyl can, of course, lead to constipation. One may consider high-fiber diet, a stool softener or a bulking agent if it is important to continue any agent that causes constipation [46].

Diarrhea is frequently seen with lithium. Slow release forms such as Lithobid result in increased lithium delivered to the colon so diarrhea may occur more frequently. Though carbamazepine rarely causes diarrhea [28], valproate may do so. As noted earlier, conversion to divalproex sodium may decrease the incidence of valproate-induced diarrhea [30].

Liver Disease

Liver disease can affect the pharmacokinetics of psychotropic agents by altering absorption, protein synthesis, biotransformation, and hepatic blood flow. Absorption of alprazolam [47] and temazepam [48] has been shown to be decreased in patients with alcoholic cirrhosis. The mechanism of this effect is unclear, but some have speculated that physical inactivity and recumbency of such patients may be responsible [47].

Albumin is decreased in cirrhosis, so the amount of a drug that is protein bound may be decreased. In addition, there is some evidence that reduced affinity of drugs for plasma proteins may occur in cirrhosis [49]. However, since psychotropic agents have a large volume of distribution, a decrease in affinity is not likely to cause a major alteration in drug effect. The explanation for this is as follows: decreased affinity results in loss of drug from the plasma compartment and thus a fall in total drug concentration. Thus, though the free *fraction* of medication is indeed increased, free drug *concentration* is largely unchanged [50].

All psychotropics (except lithium) are metabolized mainly by the liver. The principal reason for altered pharmacokinetics in liver disease is alteration of biotransformation of these agents. There are two main mechanisms of hepatic biotransformation of psychotropic agents: mixed function oxidase enzymatic oxidation and conjugation with an endogenous substrate such as glucuronic acid [50]. Hepatic enzymes which are involved in oxidation, including the cytochrome P-450 system, are strongly affected by alcoholic hepatitis, acute viral hepatitis, and active cirrhosis. Clearance of benzodiazepines metabolized by oxidation can be reduced by 1/3 to 2/3. In contrast, enzymes involved in conjugation are not affected by these diseases. Therefore, benzodiazepines metabolized by conjugation (lorazepam, oxazepam, and temazepam) are preferred with these liver diseases [11].

There is very little data on effects of liver disease on antidepressant and antipsychotic drug biotransformation. Oxidative metabolic reactions are the most important ones for the transformation of both of these groups [51, 52]. One might expect that their bioavailability would increase significantly in liver disease, since they undergo extensive first-pass metabolism when given orally [50]. However, it is important to note that this first-pass effect is with acute dosing not chronic administration.

A final pharmacokinetic issue is the reduction of hepatic blood flow that occurs in chronic cirrhosis. Drug elimination by the liver depends not only on biotransformation, but on the delivery of the drug to the liver. Blood flow reduction has a greater effect on agents such as tricyclic antidepressants which are very efficiently extracted by the liver. In contrast, clearance of drugs which are poorly extracted (e.g. benzodiazepines) is affected less by blood flow than by hepatic biotransformation [50].

There is research to suggest that some psychotropics cause more sedation in patients with cirrhosis. It would seem that metabolic considerations would be the underlying factor for this differential effect. However, it has been shown that triazolam causes more sedation in patients with chronic liver disease even when free drug concentration is the same as with controls, indicating the possibility of brain hypersensitivity [53]. In addition, chlorpromazine has been shown to cause increased EEG slowing in cirrhotics without a demonstrable difference in metabolism from controls [54]. One mechanism underlying the excess sedation in cirrhotics could be unmasking of portal systemic encephalopathy [55]. Thus, treatment of agitation in a patient with hepatic encephalopathy is often difficult. It is probably best to use haloperidol (which does not have active metabolites). Because of the potential for excess sedation, benzodiazepines would be relatively contraindicated.

Some psychotropic agents have the potential to cause liver toxicity. Carbamazepine has been estimated to cause mild asymptomatic elevations of γ-glutamyltranspeptidase (GGT), serum glutamic oxaloacetic transaminase (SGOT), and serum glutamic pyruvic transaminase (SGPT) in 5–10% of the patients [56]. Acute hepatitis, which is probably due to allergic mechanisms, had been reported to the manufacturer in only 69 persons in over 20 years of use of the medication [57]. It is essential to obtain baseline liver function tests prior to using carbamazepine and regularly thereafter, most frequently early in treatment. For a patient with underlying liver disease, carbamazepine would be relatively contraindicated. However, if it is advisable to use this medication, frequent monitoring of liver tests would be essential [56].

Valproate causes transient, mild, asymptomatic transaminase elevations in, on average, 10% of the patients. This usually occurs after 10–12 weeks of therapy. Spontaneous recovery almost always occurs; fatalities are rare. There have been cases of fatal hepatic failure due to the use of valproate, but these have generally been in children under 2 years on multiple anticonvulsants. Routine monitoring of liver tests may be advisable, especially during the first 6 months of therapy [57].

It has been known for years that chlorpromazine may cause hepatotoxicity. Mild or subclinical liver dysfunction (i.e. benign transaminase elevations) may occur in up to one-half of those who take chlorpromazine chronically. Estimates of the incidence of chlorpromazine-induced cholestatic jaundice range from 0.5 to 2.0%. It begins within 3–5 weeks after treatment is begun and is most always rapidly reversible upon discontinuation of the medication. Chronic jaundice may occur but usually resolves within a few years [58]. Though other phenothiazines may cause hepatotoxicity [59], they do so at a lower rate than chlorpromazine. Hepatic dysfunction due to non-phenothiazine neuroleptics is even rarer [51].

There are no clear guidelines for monitoring of liver function when administering neuroleptics. Levinson and Simpson [60] offer the following recommendations: (1) Asses liver function prior to and during the first 2 weeks of treatment with phenothiazines. However, it is important to realize that elevations can occur at any point during therapy. If noncholestatic disease is present, there is no increased risk of medication-induced liver damage. In patients with preexisting cholestatic liver disease, only nonphenothiazine antipsychotics should be used. In such patients, enzymes should be routinely monitored for 2 months after initiation of treatment. (2) When mild and clinically silent elevations occur, consider other etiologies first. If the medication is beneficial, one might consider continuing it (with frequent monitoring) even if it may have caused the abnormal test results. (3) The medication should be discontinued if it has caused overt hepatic dysfunction. Liver biopsy is the only way to determine definitively if cholestasis is drug-related.

Benzodiazepines, tricyclic antidepressants, phenelzine, and isocarboxazide are among others which can cause hepatotoxicity. Haloperidol causes a cholestatic reaction in less than 1% [58]. It is prudent to obtain baseline liver function studies prior to the use of any of these agents.

Parenteral Use of Psychotropics

There are two principal reasons for using psychotropic agents parenterally. First, one often uses antipsychotic and anxiolytic medications parenterally in an emergency situation. Second, there are circumstances where gastrointestinal considerations dictate that medications cannot be given by mouth. Usually such situations are temporary, e.g. a patient being unable to take anything by mouth prior to surgery. However, circumstances occasionally arise where a patient may not be allowed anything by mouth in order to rest the bowel, e.g. in severe cases of regional enteritis. The following discussion briefly addresses the parenteral use of psychotropic agents in these circumstances [for a general reference, see Baldessarini, 27].

Lorazepam, chlordiazepoxide, and diazepam may be given effectively intravenously. Only lorazepam is reliably absorbed intramuscularly. Some believe that alprazolam withdrawal is most safely done with alprazolam itself or clonazepam, which cannot be given parenterally [61]. If a patient has been taking significant doses of alprazolam and needs to abruptly stop oral intake, he/she can be placed on sublingual alprazolam. Lorazepam may also be given sublingually.

It is rarely the case that antidepressants need to be given parenterally. Usually, psychotherapy can aid in the treatment of mild depression until it is safe to resume the oral use of antidepressants. However, imipramine and amitriptyline may be used intramuscularly or intravenously. Electroconvulsive therapy should be considered for the depressed patient who cannot or will not take medications by mouth.

Neuroleptics may be needed to aid in the treatment of agitation or psychosis in patients who cannot or will not take medication by mouth. Antipsychotic medications which are available intramuscularly include chlorpromazine, fluphenazine, perphenazine, trifluoperazine, thiothixene, loxitane, and haloperidol. Currently, haloperidol is widely used intravenously, but it is not approved for use by this route. Doses often must be much higher than those given orally or intramuscularly, i.e. doses in the range of 2–10 mg every hour are commonly used. However, dosage and frequency of administration need to be adjusted to the individual situation [62].

Lithium, carbamazepine, and valproate cannot be given parenterally. For patients who are acutely manic, electroconvulsive therapy or the combination of a benzodiazepine and a neuroleptic should be tried.

References

1   Clouse RE, Lustman PJ: Psychiatric illnesses and contraction abnormalities of the esophagus. N Engl J Med 1982;309:1337–1342.
2   Bradley LA, Richter JE, Scarinci IC, Haile JM, Schan CA: Psychosocial and psychophysical assessments of patients with unexplained chest pain. Am J Med 1992;(suppl 5A):65S–73S.
3   Greenberg DB, Stern TA, Weilburg JB: The fear of choking: Three successfully treated cases. Psychosomatics 1988;29:126–129.
4   Brown SR, Schwartz JM, Summergrad, Jenike MA: Globus hystericus syndrome responsive to antidepressants. Am J Psychiatry 1986;143:917–918.

5   Clouse RE: Psychopharmacologic approaches to therapy for chest pain of presumed esophageal origin. Am J Med 1992;92(suppl 5A):106S–113S.

6   Clouse RE, Lustman PJ, Eckert TC, et al: Low-dose trazodone for symptomatic patients with esophageal contraction abnormalities. Gastroenterology 1987;92:1027–1036.

7   Nielzen S, Petterson KI, et al: The role of psychiatric factors in symptoms of hiatus hernia or gastric reflux. Acta Psychiatr Scand 1986;73:214–220.

8   Mangla JC, Pereira M: Tricyclic antidepressants in the treatment of peptic ulcer disease. Arch Intern Med 1982;142:273–275.

9   Haggerty JJ, Drossman DA: Use of psychotropic drugs in patients with peptic ulcer. Psychosomatics 1985;26:277–284.

10 Ries RK, Gilbert DA, Katon W: Tricyclic antidepressant therapy for peptic ulcer disease. Arch Intern Med 1984;144:566–569.

11 Leipzig RM: Psychopharmacology in patients with hepatic and gastrointestinal disease. Int J Psychiatry Med 1990;20:109–139.

12 Greenblatt DJ, et al: Influence of magnesium and aluminium hydroxide mixture on chlordiazepoxide absorption. Clin Pharmacol Ther 1976;19:234.

13 Greenblatt DJ, et al: Diazepam absorption: Effect of antacids and food. Clin Pharmacol Ther 1978;24:600.

14 Shader RI, et al: Steady-state plasma desmethyldiazepam during long-term clorazepate use: Effect of antacids. Clin Pharmacol Ther 1982;31:180.

15 Creelman W, Sands BF, Ciraulo, et al: Benzodiazepines; in Ciraulo DA, Shader RI, Greenblatt DJ, Creelman W (eds): Drug Interactions in Psychiatry. Baltimore, Williams & Wilkins, 1989.

16 Forrest FM, et al: Modification of chlorpromazine metabolism by some other drugs frequently administered to psychiatric patients. Biol Psychiatry 1970;2:53.

17 Henauer SA, Hollister LE: Cimetidine interaction with imipramine and nortriptyline. Clin Pharmacol Ther 1984;35:183–186.

18 Greenblatt DJ, Abernathy DR, Morse DS, et al: Clinical importance of the interaction of diazepam and cimetidine. N Engl J Med 1984;310:1039–1043.

19 Desmond PV, Patwardhan RV, et al: Cimetidine impairs elimination of chlordiazepoxide in man. Ann Intern Med 1980;93:266–268.

20 MacPhee GJ, Thompson GG, et al: Effects of cimetidine on carbamazepine auto and heteroinduction in man. Br J Clin Pharmacol 1984;18:411–419.

21 Abernethy DR, Greenblatt DJ, et al: Ranitidine does not impair oxidative or conjugative metabolism: Noninteraction with antipyrine, diazepam, and lorazepam. Clin Pharmacol Ther 1984;35:188–192.

22 Webster LK, Mihaly GW, et al: Effect of cimetidine and ranitidine on carbamazepine and sodium valproate pharmacokinetics. Eur J Clin Pharmacol 1984;27:341–343.

23 Brazer SR, Tyor MP, Pancotto FS, et al: Randomized, double-blind comparison of famotidine with ranitidine in treatment of acute, benign gastric ulcer disease. Dig Dis Sci 1989;34:1047–1052.

24 Lipsy RJ, Fennerty B, Fagan TC: Clinical review of histamine-2 receptor antagonists. Arch Intern Med 1990;150:745–751.

25 Langtry HD, Grant SM, Goa KL: Famotidine: An updated review of its pharmacokinetic properties, and therapeutic use in peptic ulcer disease and other allied diseases. Drugs 1989;38:551–590.

26 Maton PN: Omeprazole. N Engl J Med 1991;324:965–975.

27 Baldessarini RJ: Chemotherapy in Psychiatry. Cambridge, Harvard University Press, 1985.

28 Elphick M: Clinical issues in the use of carbamazepine in psychiatry: A review. Psychol Med 1989;19:591–604.

29 McElroy SL, Keck PE, Pope HG: Sodium valproate: Its use in primary psychiatric disorders. J Clin Psychopharmacol 1987;7:16–24.

30 Wilder BJ, et al: Gastrointestinal tolerance of divalproex sodium. Neurology 1983;33:808–811.

31 Wernicke JF: The side effect profile and safety of fluoxetine. J Clin Psychiatry 1985;46(3, sec 2):59–67.

32   Cole JO, Bodkin JA: Antidepressant drug side effects. J Clin Psychiatry 1990;51(1, suppl): 21–26.

33   Jenike MA, Baue L, Greist JH: Clomipramine versus fluoxetine in obsessive-compulsive disorder: A retrospective comparison of side effects and efficacy. J Clin Psychopharmacol 1990;10: 122–124.

34   Pigott TA, Pato MT, et al: Controlled comparisons of clomipramine and fluoxetine in the treatment of obsessive-compulsive disorder. Arch Gen Psychiatry 1990;47:926–932.

35   Ehrlich BE, Diamond JM: Lithium absorption: Implications for sustained-release lithium preparations (letter). Lancet 1983;i:306.

36   Wise TN: Psychological management of IBS. Pract Gastroenterol 1986;10:40–50.

37   Young SJ, Alpers DH, Norland CC: Psychiatric illness and the irritable bowel syndrome. Gasterenterologyg 1976;70:162–166.

38   Walker EA, Roy-Byrne PP, Katon WJ: Irritable bowel syndrome and psychiatric illness. Am J Psychiatry 1990;147:565–572.

39   Drossman DA, McKee DC, Sandler RS, et al: Psychosocial factors in the irritable bowel syndrome. Gasterenterology 1988;95:701–708.

40   Drossman DA, Thompson WG: The irritable bowel syndrome: Review and a graduated multicomponent treatment approach. Ann Intern Med 1992;116:1009–1016.

41   Klein KB: Controlled treatment trials in the irritable bowel syndrome: A critique. Gastroenterology 1988;95:232–241.

42   Noyes R, Cook B, et al: Reduction of gastrointestinal symptoms following treatment for panic disorder. Psychosomatics 1990;31:75–79.

43   Lydiard RB, Laraia MT, et al: Can panic disorder present as irritable bowel syndrome? J Clin Psychiatry 1986;47:470–473.

44   North CS, Clouse RE, Spitznagel EL, et al: The relation of ulcerative colitis to psychiatric factors: A review of findings and methods. Am J Psychiatry 1990;147:974–981.

45   Tarter RE, Switala J, et al: Inflammatory bowel disease: Psychiatric status of patients before and after disease onset. Int J Psychiatry Med 1987;17:173–181.

46   Taylor R: Management of constipation. 1. High fibre diets work. Br Med J 1990;300:1063–1064.

47   Juhl RP, Van Thiel DH, et al: Alprazolam pharmacokinetics in alcoholic liver disease. J Clin Pharmacol 1984;24:113–119.

48   Ochs HR, et al: Temazepam clearance unaltered in cirrhosis. Am J Gastroenterol 1986; 81:80–84.

49   Perucca E, Grimaldi R, Crema A: Interpretation of drug levels in acute and chronic disease states. Clin Pharmacokinet 1985;10:498–513.

50   Sellers EM, Bendayan R: Pharmacokinetics of psychotropic drugs in selected patient populations; in Meltzer HY (ed): Psychopharmacology: The Third Generation of Progress. New York, Raven Press, 1987, chap 146, pp 1397–1406.

51   Silver PA, Simpson GM: Antipsychotic use in the medically ill. Psychother Psychosom 1988;49: 120–136.

52   Rudorfer MV, Potter WZ: Pharmacokinetics of antidepressants; in Meltzer HY (ed): Psychopharmacology: The Third Generation of Progress. New York, Raven Press, 1987, chap 142, pp 1353–1363.

53   Bakti G, Fisch HU, et al: Mechanism of the excessive sedative response of cirrhotics to benzodiazepines: Model experiments with triazolam. Hepatology 1987;7:629–638.

54   Read AE, Laidlaw J, McCarthy CF: Effects of chlorpromazine in patients with hepatic disease. Br Med J 1969;iii:497–499.

55   Branch RA: Is there increased cerebral sensitivity to benzodiazepines in chronic liver disease? Hepatology 1987;7:773–776.

56   Stoudemire A, Moran MG, Fogel BS: Psychotropic drug use in the medically ill. Part II. Psychosomatics 1991;32:34–46.

57   Jeavons PM: Hepatotoxicity in antiepileptic drugs: Oxley J, et al (eds): Chronic Toxicity of Antiepileptic Drugs. New York, Raven Press, 1983, pp 1–46.

58   Bass NM, Ockner RK: Drug-induced liver disease; in Zakim D, Boyer TD (eds): Hepatology. Philadelphia, Saunders, 1990.

59   Jones JK, Van de Carr SW, et al: Hepatotoxicity associated with phenothiazines. Psychopharm
     Bull 1983;19:24–27.
60   Levinson DF, Simpson GM: Serious nonextrapyramidal adverse effects of neuroleptics: Sudden
     death, agranulocytosis and hepatotoxicity; in Meltzer HY (ed): Psychopharmacology: The
     Third Generation of Progress. New York, Raven Press, 1987, chap 150, pp 1431–1436.
61   Herman JB, Rosenbaum JF, Brotman AW: The alprazolam to clonazepam switch for the treat-
     ment of panic disorder. J Clin Psychopharmacol 1987;175–178.
62   Tesar GE, Stern TA: Evaluation and treatment of agitation in the intensive care unit. J Intens
     Care Med 1986;1:137–148.

Steven A. Epstein, MD, Department of Psychiatry, Georgetown University Medical Center,
3800 Reservoir Road, NW, Washington, DC 20007–2197 (USA)

Silver PA (ed): Psychotropic Drug Use in the Medically Ill.
Adv Psychosom Med. Basel, Karger, 1994, vol 21, pp 61–89

Use of Psychotropic Medication in the Neurologically Ill

Anton Trinidad, Paul A. Silver[1]

Department of Psychiatry, Georgetown University, Washington, D. C., USA

The expanding use of psychotropic medication in clinical practice has made the boundary between neurology and psychiatry more fluid with a wider area of overlap than ever before. Neurological diseases, such as Huntington's disease, multiple sclerosis and Parkinson's disease often produce a host of psychiatric symptoms and sequelae which are amenable to psychopharmacotherapy. It is common to find patients with these diseases under the care of both a neurologist and a psychiatrist. Integration will continue apace as more biologic correlates of psychiatric symptoms are identified in both psychiatric and neurologic illnesses. Maintaining thorough knowledge of the pharmacology of psychotropic medications in these patients is necessary for both neurologists and psychiatrists to provide comprehensive, competent treatment.

This paper will provide a review of the use of psychotropic agents in neurologic diseases with psychiatric manifestations, as well as those in which the neurologic condition complicates the pharmacotherapy of comorbid psychiatric illness.

General Principles

The clinician contemplating pharmacotherapy in a patient whose brain is compromised by a disease process or injury is walking a risk/benefit tightrope. In addition to having pathology which often sensitizes the central nervous sys-

[1] We would like to thank Kit Strauss, Susan Weigert, and Rochelle Silver for their assistance in the preparation of this manuscript.

tem to all effects of psychotropics, the neurologically ill patient is oftentimes generally debilitated. Dehydration, protein-calorie malnutrition, secondary infections, and cognitive and/or motor impairments may compromise compliance and alter absorption, distribution and elimination of psychotropic medications.

Lipid affinity is one of the most crucial factors in determining the rate at which a drug enters the brain. Under normal conditions, lipophilic drugs with high partition coefficients (the ratio of solubity in olive oil to water) reach high concentrations in the brain quickly while nonlipophilic drugs may never enter the brain due to exclusion by the blood-brain barrier. However, in a study assessing blood-brain barrier permeability in subjects with craniocerebral injuries, a direct relationship between permeability (as measured by CSF albumin/IgG ratio) and severity of injury was found [1]. Other studies show that changes in the ingetrity of the blood-brain barrier alter the transport of foreign molecules to the brain [2]. Equally crucial is the role of the choroid plexus in the elimination of substances from the brain [3]. Inflammatory conditions like choriomeningitis or encephalitis thus effect both the entrance and exit of pharmacotherapeutic drugs to and from the brain and may provide scenarios for central toxicity. Not much data are presently available to give clinicians precise guidance regarding dosage in these cases except the venerable principle of giving the lowest effective dose.

A review of the pharmacologic actions of psychotropics is far beyond the scope of this paper, but knowledge of these actions is imperative to the practice of competent pharmacotherapy. For the reader unfamiliar with this information, we refer you to Rubey and Lydiard's paper in this volume, or a basic psychopharmacology text.

Seizure Disorder

Comorbid seizure and psychiatric disorders present a challenge to the clinician because of the frequency of coexistance of these conditions [4] and the epileptogenic potential of many psychotropics. We will focus on the use of traditional psychotropics in the epileptic; the expanding use of anticonvulsants for psychiatric illness will not be discussed.

Antipsychotics

There is controversy regarding the effects of various antipsychotics on seizure threshold. Findings in numerous clinical and basic pharmacologic studies are often at odds. Tedeschi et al. [5] measured the effect of six phenothiazines on the minimal electroshock seizure threshold in mice, finding that chlorpromazine, in moderate doses, lowered the threshold while having no effect in high or low doses. Trifluoperazine had little effect on seizure threshold and perchlorperazine increased it. Using a similar model, Chen's group [6] found that several antipsychotics, including chlorpromazine, trifluoperazine and haloperidol, lowered the seizure threshold in low doses but raised it in high doses.

The action of antipsychotics on the spike activity of perfused guinea pig hippocampal slices was studied by Oliver et al. [7] who found that chlorpromazine and thioridazine increased spiking at low concentrations but that this activity decreased at high concentrations. Conversely, haloperidol and fluphenazine caused greater increases in spiking at higher concentrations, though the curve flattened out at the highest concentrations, with haloperidol being more provocative than fluphenazine. Pimozide caused a slight increase in spiking at low levels and molindone caused no changes.

Itil [8] found that, among antipsychotics, chlorpromazine had the most significant effect on the EEG. Thioridazine had somewhat less of an effect. Trifluoperazine and fluphenazine caused the least amount of epileptiform activity of all phenothiazines and no seizures were observed in patients on fluphenazine. Haloperidol produced fewer disturbances than did thiothixene or fluphenazine, but the doses of Haldol used were much lower (15 mg for haloperidol vs. 80 mg for the others). This may have been an important factor considering the dose-related effect of Haldol on guinea pig hippocampus. Molindone caused less dysrhythmia than did trifluoperazine. Seizures did not occur in patients treated with thiothixene or molindone [8].

Several clinical reviews [9–11] implicate chlorpromazine as the antipsychotic most likely to provoke seizures. Unlike findings in the animal studies, clinical experience indicates that high or rapidly increased doses of chlorpromazine are more commonly epileptogenic [9, 11].

Given these discrepancies, it is hard to give clear guidance in the choice of antipsychotic for patients at risk for seizures. Though researchers have, at various times, proposed that more anticholinergic and less dopamine-blocking agents may be the safest [12], the evidence does not support this [7]. Indeed, chlorpromazine, which meets these putative criteria for safety, is the agent most commonly cited to provoke seizures. Clozapine, a weak dopamine blocker with significant anticholinergic effects is particularly epileptogenic, especially when used in high doses [13]. Conversely, thioridazine, with a pharmacologic profile similar to chlorpromazine, seems relatively benign [11, 14]. The sedative potential of a medication, which some proposed as being correlated with ability to provoke seizures [11], cannot be used as a guide since the three most sedating antipsychotics, clozapine, thioridazine and chlorpromazine differ in epileptogenic potential.

Nonetheless, some conclusions can be drawn. Chlorpromazine should not be used in patients at risk for seizures. Clozapine should be avoided unless the potential benefits of this novel antipsychotic clearly outweigh the real possibility of its causing seizures in the vulnerable patient. Haloperidol should be used with caution since the study which indicated it as innocuous utilized low doses [8] and there is animal evidence that epileptogenic potential increases with dose [7]. Of note is the report of a patient who developed complex-partial status epilepticus when his daily dose of haloperidol was raised from 50 to 100 mg [15]. There is consensus from the basic and clinical literature that molindone is relatively safe in this population [7, 8, 11, 16]. Several authorities have proposed that thioridazine and fluphenazine are also safe [11, 14, 16], but there is less evidence to support this.

In addition to the choice of medication, it is vital, when medicating patients at risk for seizuring, to minimize other factors which may lower the seizure threshold, to use the lowest doses of antipsychotic possible and to increase doses slowly [10–12]. In patients with a known seizure disorder, care should be taken that anticonvulsant levels are adequate and levels must be monitored since antipsychotics have been found to both raise and lower levels throught their competition for hepatic enzymes [12]. Patients who develop seizures on antipsychotics should be thoroughly evaluated for underlying neurologic disease [11] and the onset of focal seizures should raise a high index of suspicion for the presence of a structural lesion [10].

Antidepressants
Unlike the antipsychotics, where the different chemical classes can be considered together, different types of antidepressants have varying effects on the seizure threshold and there can be disparity within a class. Tricyclics differ in their effects on seizure threshold. There is evidence that imipramine, clomipramine, amitriptyline, and nortriptyline all increase the risk of seizuring in the susceptible patient [11, 14, 17–19]. Clomipramine may be particularly hazardous; a survey described by Edwards [2] shows that seizures were reported in patients taking clomipramine with a frequency out of proportion to its market share. A study of the literature by Burley [21] cited by Trimble [18] indicated that clomipramine was associated with a 3% incidence of seizures compared to a 0.7% incidence for imipramine, though his study has been criticized on methodologic grounds [18, 22]. Desipramine and trimipramine may be somewhat less likely to cause seizures [14], though seizures have been reported with the use of these agents [23, 24]. It should be noted that in a review of overdoses by Wedin et al. [25], desipramine caused a higher frequency of seizures than did other tricyclics. Conversely, there have been reports of the use of imipramine as an anticonvulsant in absence and in minor motor seizures [26–28].

Among the tricyclics, doxepin is thought to be relatively safe for use in the epileptic population [14], though Ojemann et al. [29] reported an increase in seizure frequency in 3 of 32 patients treated with doxepin. In an earlier study, Ojemann et al. [30] found that doxepin improved seizure control in 15 of 19 epileptics, worsened control in 2 and caused no change in 2. Other researchers found that doxepin, at higher concentrations, lowered spiking in perfused guinea pig hippocampal slices [31]. Simeon et al. [32] injected normal volunteers with imipramine, doxepin, chlordiazepoxide and diazepam and found that doxepin had an effect on the EEG closer to that of the anticonvulsant diazepam than of imipramine [32].

It is interesting to note that protriptyline and trimipramine are even better at suppressing spiking than is doxepin, but that clinically, they have a higher association with seizuring [14, 29].

Given the conflicting data, it is hard to come to firm conclusions, but the evidence seems to support the use of doxepin when a tricyclic is needed in a patient at risk for seizuring. If doxepin's high sedative, anticholinergic and α-adrenergic blocking properties preclude its use, and a tricyclic is required, desipramine may be an alternative. Imipramine, amitriptyline and clomipramine should be avoided. As with using the antipsychotics, low doses should be initiated and raised in small, slow increments to the lowest dose which has the desired effect. In the patient with a known seizure disorder, adequate anticonvulsant levels must be maintained. Preskorn and Fast [33] found that seizuring is often related to high tricyclic levels so antidepressant levels must also be monitored. Keep in mind that anticonvulsants can lower tricyclic levels (except for clonazepam which may increase them) and that tricyclics can change anticonvulsant levels [14, 16]. In addition, carbemazepine is a tricyclic, so there can be synergism in regard to side effects [14].

Monoamine oxidase inhibitors (MAOIs) may be of use in depressed patients at risk for seizuring. Chen et al. [6] found that tranylcypromine increases extensor seizure threshold in mice [6] and other MAOIs were found to be anticonvulsant in animal models [34]. The above-noted survey reported by Edwards [20] failed to show greater than expected seizuring in patients on MAOIs. Several reviews have endorsed the monoamine oxidase inhibitors as being relatively safe for use in patients at risk for seizures [11, 14, 16].

Several of the 'newer' antidepressants have been reported to have high epileptogenic potential. Maprotiline, a tetracyclic, was found to cause an enormous number of seizures despite a relatively small market share [20]. In overdose, maprotiline was more likely to cause seizures than the tricyclics [25]. Although these frequencies are much higher than those reported in other surveys, under reporting may be a factor in this discrepancy as may be the relatively short duration of monitoring in the premarketing period [35]. In their study of maprotiline-associated seizures, Dessain et al. [35] found that, in a sample of patients whose seizures were reported to the manufacturer, 42% of the seizures occurred after 6 weeks of treatment. When this sample was combined with 11 patients at their own institution, it was found that 68% of the patients were treated with doses which were above the recommended 225 mg/day limit or had their doses increased faster than the manufacturer's guidelines dictated. The authors note that despite the high doses used in 11 patients at their hospital, their plasma levels were on the low side. This, combined with the frequency of late-onset seizures while on a stable dose of medication, led Dessain's group to postulate the accumulation of an epileptogenic metabolite as the cause of seizures. Maprotiline should not be used in any patient with a seizure disorder or at risk for seizuring. The manufacturer's guidlines regarding dose escalation and maximum dose should be strictly adhered to for all patients.

Bupropion, a novel, monocyclic antidepressant, was temporarily withdrawn from the market shortly after its release when it was reported to have precipitated seizures in 4 non-depressed bulimic patients in a study of 55 such subjects [36]. Several other reviews failed to reveal incidences near the 7.3% found in that study. In premarketing trials involving 2,400 patients, the incidence of seizures in patients taking less than 450 mg/day was 0.3%, while those taking 450–600 mg/day or greater than 600 mg/day were 2.3 and 2.8%, respectively [37]. In a subsequent prospective study in which 1986 subjects completed 8 weeks of treatment with up to 450 mg of bupropion and 1,616 went on to a continuation phase, only 0.24% of the patients had seizures during the initial 8 weeks with a seizure rate of 0.40% reported for the entire study period [37]. Davidson [38] reported on 37 patients who seizured out of a total of 4,262 subjects treated with bupropion. The seizure rate for those taking greater than 450 mg/day was 2.19% while that for subjects taking lower doses was 0.44%. In a literature review comparing seizure rates in patients being treated with imipramine, amitriptyline or bupropion, Peck et al. [22] found only 1 patient of 801 taking 450 mg/day or less of bupropion seizured, and that patient had a history of seizure disorder. The incidence of seizures at doses between 500 and 750 mg/day was 0.85% in patients with no known predisposition to seizuring. These rates compared favorably with those for imipramine. It is interesting to note that the elderly may have a somewhat decreased frequency of seizuring on bupropion [37–39].

Thus, when used according to the current recommendations not to exceed a daily dose of 450 mg or to give greater than 150 mg per dose, it appears that bupropion is no more epileptogenic than the tricyclics as a group. It should probably be avoided in patients with a history of bulimia, but may be of use in the elderly. Indeed, it may have been the relatively young ages of the bulimic patients that put them at risk for seizuring. There are really no data which would help ascertain if bupropion is more likely to precipitate seizures in at risk individual than are other agents. Since there are agents which are less epileptogenic, bupropion should probably be avoided in this population unless it is the only agent to which a patient has been found to respond.

Amoxapine is a metabolite of loxapine which possesses antidepressant and antipsychotic activity. In a review of overdoses occurring over an 18-month period, amoxapine caused seizures in 36.4% of the 33 patients who overdosed, compared to a 4.3% seizure rate in the 446 patients who overdosed on other cyclic antidepressants [40]. There have also been reports of irreversible neurological damage in patients who have had multiple seizures after amoxapine overdoses [41]. In the light of these reports, amoxapine should be avoided in patients at risk for seizuring.

There have been case reports of seizures in patients on trazodone [42–44]. Two of the three seizures reported were in patients with pretreatment EEG abnormalities [43, 44] and Lefkowitz et al. [43] note that the 30 patients whose seizures were reported to the manufacturer all had risk factors for seizuring. There are not enough data to compare the seizure rate for trazodone with those of other agents.

Despite its wide use, there have been few reports of seizures in patients taking fluoxetine. Ware and Stewart [45] describe a patient with pretreatment epileptiform activity on EEG who had a seizure after 3 days on fluoxetine 20 mg/day. They note that the patient had a 0.5-mg/day dose of alprazolam discontinued 10 days before the seizure. In a review of 1,378 subjects treated with fluoxetine, one person was reported to have two definite seizures after an overdose of 3,000 mg of fluoxetine [46]. Four other subjects were suspected of having seizures, but these were not confirmed. Cooper's [47] 1988 review of clinical trials found only three reports of definite seizures, one following an overdose, one in a patient with a history of petit mal who actually had a decrease in seizure frequency and one in a 71-year-old patient without predisposing factors. Other reported cases were of patients who were on concomitant medications [48, 49] or had CNS lesions [50]. There is some evidence from animal studies that fluoxetine might raise the seizure threshold [51, 52]. Given the pausity of reports of seizures despite extensive use of fluoxetine, and the animal work which indicates its possibly positive effect on the seizure threshold, fluoxetine may prove to be a safe agent to use in patients at risk for seizuring. Fluoxetine and its metabolite's long half-lives and their propensity to effect the metabolism and blood levels of other agents necessitate caution using it with, or before, other agents. Though, as of yet, little has been written about the epileptogenic potentials of sertraline and paroxetine, neither agent seems particularly hazardous in this regard.

Psychostimulants are coming into increased use in the elderly and medically ill. Wroblewski et al. [53] note that the Physicians' Desk Reference claims that methylphenidate may lower the seizure threshold [54]. Wroblewski's group cites studies in which stimulants were safely used in epileptics [55–57] and in their retrospective review of 30 brain-injured patients with posttraumatic seizures, they found the use of methylphenidate increased seizure frequency in 4 patients, while it reduced the frequency in 13 and caused no change in 13 [53]. Thus, it seems that psychostimulants can be used with caution in at-risk patients.

Rosenstein et al. [58] in a review of antidepressant-associated seizures, found that a 'significant proportion' of such seizures occur in patients with predisposing factors, including withdrawal states and multiple concomitant medications. Safe use of antidepressants requires the appropriate management of these other conditions, and, as noted above, adequate coverage with anticonvulsants when indicated.

Though electroconvulsive therapy (ECT) produces generalized seizures, the effect of these seizures is to raise the seizure threshold [59]. Sackheim et al. [59] report on the cessation of seizuring in a 19-year-old woman with intractable epilepsy during a course of ECT. Both Sackheim's paper and Abrams' textbook on ECT [60] cite reports of the use of ECT to treat epilepsy. ECT can be used to treat psychiatric illness in the seizure-disordered patient and may ameliorate the psychosis which can be associated with epilepsy [60]. Anticonvulsants should be continued during the ECT, though they will increase the electrical dose needed to produce seizures [60]. There does not seem to be an increase in spontaneous seizures following ECT [61].

Benzodiazepines are anticonvulsants and are, thus, safe to use in patients with seizure disorders. However, caution must be used when discontinuing or tapering these agents, since these actions may produce seizuring, especially in the vulnerable patient [11]. Buspirone, a non-benzodiazepine anxiolytic, has not been reported to produce seizuring or change the seizure threshold. The caveat warning against the abrupt discontinuation of benzodiazepines also holds when switching to buspirone; the benzodiazepine has to be tapered.

Jefferson et al. [62] reviewed the reports of the use of lithium in seizure disorder patients. Though there have been some reports of increased seizure frequency with lithium use, most papers indicate a reduction or no change in seizure frequency in most patients. There is some evidence from animal studies which indicates that the site of the seizure focus may determine whether lithium increases or decreases the seizure threshold [63]. Given the mounting evidence that two anticonvulsants, carbamazepine and valproic acid, may be used as alternatives to lithium in bipolar disorders, it might be prudent to choose one of these agents for use in the bipolar patient with a seizure disorder.

Dementia

The prescribing of psychotropic drugs for patients with dementia is widespread. However, studies to evaluate the efficacy of such medications in demented patients have often been methodologically limited. Nevertheless, the sheer magnitude of the behavioral, cognitive and psychosocial problems produced by dementing illnesses calls for constant reassessments of the specific roles which pharmacotherapy can play in the management of patients with these problems.

It is vital, when considering pharmacotherapy in the demented elderly, to have a detailed understanding of the pharmacokinetic changes that occur with aging, in addition to appreciating the altered responses of the impaired brain to drugs. Absorption, distribution, metabolism and excretion are all affected by aging [64]. Furthermore, there is a high frequency of concurrent medical illness, with the attendant physiologic changes as well as the potential for drug interactions. For a fuller discussion of this area, we refer you to the paper by Rubey and Lydiard in this volume.

Before embarking on drug treatment, it is crucial to identify and correct those things which may worsen the symptoms of dementia, such as metabolic abnormalities and the administration of anticholinergic medications. The clinician must also be certain that he/she is dealing with dementia and not a reversible, though potentially life-threatening, delirium. The discussion which follows assumes that the patient has had a thorough neurological and medical evaluation which has ruled-out treatable causes of cognitive changes. Finally, one must always attend to the nonpharmacologic interventions which are helpful to the demented patient.

Of particular relevance in the pharmacotherapy of dementia is the concept of targeting symptoms for treatment. Reports on psychotropic drug use in nursing homes estimate the prevalence of use from 37 to 75% [65, 66]. Despite these high figures, the indications for their use varies widely and have included agitation, behavioral dyscontrol, psychosis and aggression. To date, few studies have been helpful in delineating which symptoms of dementia respond best to which psychotropics. Two double-blind studies have generated some data on the efficacy of neuroleptics in certain behavioral disturbances in the elderly [67, 68], but in these studies not all subjects were diagnosed with dementia. That neuroleptics can be efficacious in alleviating psychosis seen in demented patients has been shown by some, but not all, studies [69–72]. The evidence for nonpsychotic agitation and other nonspecific behavioral disturbances benefiting from pharmacotherapy is less clear. Benzodiazepines, barbiturates and meprobamate have been used for behavioral control, but their utility has been limited by troublesome side effects such as ataxia and oversedation [66, 73,

74]. Greendyke and Kanter [75] used the beta-blocker pindolol in a double-blind study with 11 demented patients and found that the target symptoms of hostility, uncooperativeness and repetitive behavior responded best to this treatment with optimal dosages being 40–60 mg daily. No significant hypotension or bradycardia were seen. Propranolol has also been utilized in the treatment of agitation in dementia [76]. There is some evidence that the antidepressant trazodone may help ameliorate agitation in demented patients, even in the absence of depression [77].

The use of antidepressant medication in dementia is often complicated by troublesome adverse reactions including postural hypotension, cardiac conduction delay and anticholinergic effects. This is unfortunate since depression may complicate dementia and the elderly are at particular risk for suicide [78]. The most frequent initial choice of antidepressant medication is a heterocyclic agent though the use of newer agents is becoming more common. Though various tricyclics are equally efficacious in most cases of depression [79], it is prudent, in the elderly, to use a secondary amine due to its lower incidence and severity of side effects. Nortriptyline is the tricyclic least prone to cause orthostasis and desipramine the least anticholinergic. Monoamine oxidase inhibitors (MAOI) may have a place in treating depressed, demented patients. They are relatively free of anticholinergic effects and do not effect the cardiac conduction system, but can cause severe orthostasis.

Experience with the use of later-generation antidepressants like fluoxetine, buproprion, sertraline, and paroxetine is still limited and, though they appear relatively safe, they should be used with caution. Psychostimulants have been reported efficacious in medically ill patients [80, 81] but await further evaluation in dementia.

ECT may be considered for depression complicating dementia especially in the presence of concurrent medical illnesses which preclude pharmacologic trials. ECT may transiently worsen existing deficits but depression itself can worsen cognition and the use of ECT may cause a net improvement [82–84].

Parkinson's Disease

Although motor signs are prominent in Parkinson's disease, psychiatric comorbidity, in the forms of depression, dementia and psychosis, is common. The prevalence of depression in Parkinson's is between 20 and 63 % [85]. Dementia increases with the progression of the disease and psychosis may result from the disease process itself or as an adverse consequence of dopamimetic therapy.

There does not seem to be a clear relationship between mood and motor symptoms in Parkinson's. Depression appears to be more common in patients who have the dopamine-responsive symptoms of bradykinesia and rigidity and increases during the 'off' periods in patients who display the 'on-off' phenomenon [86]. Huber et al. [87] found a correlation between the severity of disease and dementia, but neither were related to depression.

Parkinson's patients are more depressed than similarly disabled patients with other conditions [88, 89]. Thus, it appears that depression is a manifestation of the basic disease process and not simply a response to a distressing illness. Similarly, the dementia represents brain disease, and not cognitive fogging related to depression.

In his review of the literature, Cummings [86] found few reports of antidepressant effects for most treatments for Parkinsons's [86]. Anticholinergics may cause a mild euphoria. Some studies indicate that *l*-dopa may have little effect on [90], or may even worsen [91], depression. Bromocriptine, in high doses, may decrease depression [92]. The monoamine oxidase B inhibitor, selegiline, is used to potentiate *l*-dopa [93] and retards the progression of the disease, perhaps by preventing the formation of hydroxyl radicals [86, 94]. In the relatively low doses used to treat parkinsonism, selegiline has, at most, a nominal antidepressant effect [95].

Heterocyclic antidepressants may be used with or without antiparkinson medications. Imipramine, nortriptyline and desipramine can be effective in relieving depression [96–98] and, in some studies [96, 97], imipramine and desipramine have reduced parkinsonian symptoms. However, the antiparkinsonian effects do not always correlate with the antidepressant effects. Among the heterocyclics, amoxapine, with its dopamine-blocking activity, should be avoided. Driver [99] cites a report of doxepine causing parkinsonian side effects.

Because of their ability to block the presynaptic reuptake of dopamine, there hase been particular interest in the use of nomifensin and bupropion in patients with Parkinson's, both as antidepressants and as possible treatments for the movement disorder. Nomifensin, which was taken off the market in the United States because of its propensity to cause hemolytic anemia, was of modest, if any, help in relieving parkinsonian symptoms [100–102]. Only Bedard's group monitored depression in their subjects and found that neither of the two clinically depressed patients showed improvement in mood. Nonetheless, all three papers advocated the use of nomifensin in depressed Parkinson's patients.

Goetz et al. [103] used bupropion in 18 patients with Parkinson's, 12 of whom were depressed. The patients were taking *l*-dopa and trihexyphenidyl, but not bromocriptine. Ten patients showed improvement in their parkinsonism, but only 5 of the 12 depressed patients got better. Changes in depression and parkinsonian symptoms were independent of one another. Three patients suffered from increased psychosis and one had a worsening of dyskinesia. A report of delirium in a 75-year-old patient with Parkinson's concurrently taking amantadine and bupropion sounds a cautionary note [104].

The limited utility of dopamine reuptake blockers makes sense since they rely on the production of dopamine in intact dopaminergic neurons to produce their effect. Other indirect dopamine agonists, such as amphetamine and methylphenidate, which cause increased dopamine release, are of limited use in Parkinson's for either the movement disorder [105] or depression [106]. Cantello et al. [106] showed that depressed Parkinson's patients had a blunting of the euphorogenic effect of methylphenidate. Nondepressed Parkinson's patients did not show this blunting, indicating a possible role for the degeneration of the mesolimbic dopaminergic tracts in the genesis of parkinsonian depression. It is interesting to note that depressed, non-Parkinson's patients did not show a blunted response to methylphenidate.

Caley and Friedman [107] reviewed reports of fluoxetine-induced parkinsonian symptoms and found that 3 of the 5 patients described were taking haloperidol or lithium. They then reviewed the records of 23 patients with Parkinson's disease who were treated with up to 40 mg/day of fluoxetine. Only 3 patients had a worsening of their parkinsonism and 2 improved. The authors note that their patients were taking antiparkinsonian medication which may have protected them from the effects of fluoxetine. Although the concomitant use of fluoxetine and *l*-deprenyl did not produce the 'serotonin syndrome' in this series, which is consistant with the metabolism of serotonin by MAO-A, there has been a report of a patient developing diaphoresis and hypertension while taking *l*-deprenyl 5 mg with fluoxetine, bromocriptine and *l*-dopa/carbidopa [108]. In addition, Montastruc et al. [109] describe a patient who developed intermittent hypertension with elevated catecholamines while being treated with *l*-deprenyl 10 mg and fluoxetine. Though Caley and Friedman's [107] review appears to indicate that fluoxetine can be used safely in most patients with Parkinson's disease, Steur [110] reports 4 patients whose parkinsonism worsened while on fluoxetine but returned to baseline after the drug was discontinued. Clearly, prospective double-blind studies are still needed.

Though there is an extensive literature on the use of MAO-B inhibitors in patients with Parkinson's disease, little has been written on the use of traditional, irreversible, mixed A and B MAOIs. This is probably due to the fact that MAOIs cannot be used with *l*-dopa for fear of precipitating a hypertensive crisis. There is, however, one report of a patient being successfully treated with a combination of phenelzine and amantadine [111].

There is some evidence that GABA agonists may exert prodomaminergic and antidopaminergic effects depending on dose [112]. However, there have been some reports of benzodiazepines worsening parkinsonian symptoms [113]. Buspirone, a non-benzodiazepine anxiolytic with possible dopaminergic agonist effects, does not relieve the symptoms of Parkinson's disease in usual antianxiety doses. High doses worsen parkinsonism, but reduce treatment-emergent dyskinesias [113].

There are several roles for ECT in the treatment of patients with Parkinson's disease. Both depression and movement disorder can respond to ECT [114]. Treatment responses are independent, with some patients having amelioration of either type of symptom or of both [115, 116]. In their review, Atre-Vaidya and Jambala [115] found that when the depression predates the motor signs, both the movement disorder and depression respond to ECT [114, 117]. When motor manifestations come first, often they, but not the depression, will respond to ECT [115, 118]. There have also been reports of psychosis [119] and mania [115] resolving with the use of ECT in this population. ECT has been used in patients with movement disorder alone with good results and may be of particular use in the patients who develop the 'on-off' phenomena after long-term use of dopamimetics [120, 121], though one group did not find it to be effective [122].

The duration of response to ECT ranges from 2 to 41 weeks [120]. Since improvement may be short-lived, there may be a role for maintenance ECT. It is thought that the mechanism of action of ECT is to increase the sensitization of dopamine receptors [116, 120, 121], thus dyskinesias may be made worse by ECT [116, 117]. Patients with Parkinson's disease, especially when complicated by dementia, may be vulnerable to increased confusion during ECT [123] which may be diminished by lowering the dose of dopaminergic drugs prior to treatment [124]. The presence of dementia may be a poor prognostic sign for the improvement of depression [115, 118] though Douyon's group thought that older patients were more responsive to ECT than younger ones [116].

Other than in patients with a pre-existing bipolar disorder, mania is rare in untreated Parkinson's disease, but it may complicate the use of dopamimetic agents [85, 125]. In some cases, drug-induced mania will respond to a lowering of dose or switching to another agent. Little has been written about the use of mood stabilizers such as lithium, carbemazepine or valproic acid in parkinsonian patients. There is no clear contraindication to their use in Parkinson's patients with ideopathic mania or in those with drug-induced mania whose parkinsonian symptoms break through on lowered doses of anti-Parkinson's drugs. There is some evidence that lithium may be effective in reducing the 'on-off' phenomenon in patients undergoing chronic *l*-dopa therapy [126]. When treatment emergent mania is accompanied by psychosis, the manic symptoms may respond to an antipsychotic. As noted above, manic symptoms may also respond to ECT [115].

Psychosis and hallucinosis can occur in the natural course of Parkinson's disease, but are more commonly a complication of treatment [85, 91]. *l*-dopa therapy tends to worsen psychosis [90] so it is not a treatment for psychosis complicating the natural course of the disease. Indeed, amantadine, anticholinergics and dopamine agonists such as bromocriptine and lergotril can all be psychomimetic [127]. When hallucinations and/or delusions arise, the first step should be to decrease all antiparkinsonian medications to the lowest doses which allow the patient to maintain mobility and activities of daily living [91, 127]. If this does not control the psychosis, a careful trial of low doses of antipsychotics may be undertaken [85, 128]. Clozapine, a novel antipsychotic which causes minimal extrapyramidal effects [129], has been used in low doses (12.5–200 mg/day) with good results to treat psychosis in patients with Parkinson's without worsening the movement disorder [130, 131]. Sedation, orthostasis, potent anticholinergic effects and sialorrhea are common side effects of clozapine and can complicate its use in this population [131, 132]. Other considerations are clozapine's extraordinarily high price and its tendency to cause agranulocytosis in 1–2% of the users; this latter feature leading to the requirement of weekly white blood cell counts. As noted above, ECT is another treatment option for psychosis in parkinsonian patients [119].

Huntington's Disease

Huntington's disease (HD) is an autosomal-dominant syndrome causing choreoathetotic movement disorder, dementia, and, frequently, affective disorders, psychosis, agitation and personality changes [133]. The onset of symptoms is most often in the fourth and fifth decades but has been reported to occur as early as age 4 [134] and as late as 75 years [135]. The locus for the HD gene has been found on chromosome 4 [136]. The diagnosis is usually made when choreoathetotic movements develop in a patient with a positive family history; spontaneous mutations are rare. Psychiatric symptoms, such as affective disorder, may precede the onset of movement disorder by up to 20 years [137], and are often the major cause of disability in Huntington's patients [138]. Caudate nucleus hypometabolism and atrophy are usually found [133] as are decreases in γ-aminobutyric acid (GABA) and glutamic acid decarboxylase [139]. The interval between onset of symptoms and death is 10–30 years.

Though some of the behavioral and motor manifestations of HD can be palliated with agents that reduce dopamine transmission, such as antipsychotics and tetrabenazines, there is little evidence that the overall course of the disease is modified [140]. Antidopaminergics can cause extrapyramidal side effects [141, 142] and have variable, modest effects on psychosis [138]. There have been some reports which indicate that clozapine may reduce psychiatric symptoms in Huntington's patients without causing extrapyramidal effects [142, 143] but without improving the movement disorder [143].

Vegetative symptoms of depression may be reduced by the use of tricyclic antidepressants, but symptoms such as hopelessness [138] and apathy [144] are resistant to treatment. The anticholinergic properties of these agents can worsen the movement disorder [139, 144] and may limit their use. The non-anticholinergic MAOIs [145] and ECT [133] have been used successfully in these patients and there may be an, as of yet, unsubstantiated role for the use of non-tricyclic selective serotonin reuptake blockers.

Irritability, agitation, and explosive behavior are major management problems in patients with HD. β-Blockers have been used with some success [146], but can cause paradoxical worsening [147, 148]. In a small study using lithium and haloperidol, both alone and in combination, the administration of the drugs together reduced irritability and aggressive outburts [149]. Of note is the finding that the use of haloperidol alone caused an increase in depression. Though bipolar disorders were found in 9% of the patients in a survey of HD patients in Maryland [137], little has been written about the treatment of mania in this population. Despite the fact that the GABA system seems to be involved in the pathophysiology of HD, pharmacologic manipulation of this system seems to be of little consistent help [139, 150].

Multiple Sclerosis

Psychiatric disturbances are frequent in patients with multiple sclerosis (MS) with mood disorders being the most common. Cognitive deterioration and psychotic episodes tend to be seen in the later stages of the illness. In reviewing studies of MS patients, Petersen and Kokmen [151] found that certain cognitive functions like memory and conceptual processing are preferentially impaired. It is not uncommon for MS to be initially diagnosed as an idiopathic or primary psychiatric disorder [152]. Furthermore, the treatment of MS often involves the use of steroids and ACTH which, in and of themselves, give rise to various psychopathologic states and behavioral disturbances termed, perhaps too loosely, 'steroid psychosis'. Reports of steroid-induced panic attacks have also appeared in the literature [153].

No systematic study of antipsychotic use in patients with MS has, to our knowledge, been done. When psychosis occurs, an attempt must be made to determine whether steroids are the cause and, if so, taper the hormones if neurologically feasible. Antipsychotics can be given, but extreme care should be used in cases where muscular spasticity could potentially be worsened by dystonia precipitated by the use of a high potency agent. The use of lower potency agents or prophylactic antiparkinsonian agents should be considered in these cases. Despite the overall lack of specific guidelines that are empirically based for the use of antipsychotics in MS, they may provide significant symptom alleviation when psychosis is clearly present. Rudick et al. [154] write that antipsychotic use in MS is not different from their use in the general psychiatric population [154].

The depression that occurs in MS is generally moderately severe in its magnitude [155]. Both neurobiological impairment and psychogenic reactivity to the disease itself have been implicated in the depression seen in MS [156]. Depression appears to be more common in MS patients with cerebral involvement than in those with primarily spinal cord disease [154]. It is difficult to evaluate the efficacy of treatment modalities due to the protean manifestations of the illness and the relapsing-remitting nature of its symptoms.

One double-blind placebo-controlled study used desipramine in doses up to 200 mg/day in patients with MS diagnosed with major depression [157]. Of 28 patients, 14 received desipramine for 5 weeks and the other 14 received placebo plus individual psychotherapy. Significant improvements were seen in the desipramine group compared to the placebo group on the Hamilton Depression Rating Scale. In this study, side effects significantly limitated the attainment of target therapeutic blood levels. The authors speculated that the usual range of therapeutic levels for desipramine may not apply to MS patients, which in turn may imply that the drug distribution kinetics may be different in MS.

To date, little has been written about the use of fluoxetine, bupropion, sertaline, or paroxetine in patients with MS. Their more benign side effect profiles make them seem like attractive alternatives to the heterocyclics and MAOIs. Though Flax et al. [158] reported good responses with minimal side effects in 20 MS patients treated with fluoxetine, there have been anecdotal reports which raise the possibility that fluoxetine may precipitiate MS exacerbations [159].

Emotional lability, sometimes manifested as pathological laughing and weeping, may occur in MS and may be quite distressing. Amitriptyline has been used successfully in some cases [154, 160]. Other tricyclics may also be effective as are *l*-dopa or bromocriptine [154]. Manic symptoms have been noted in association with MS [161]. The use of thymoleptics like lithium or carbamazepine in these cases remain uninvestigated in a systematized fashion. George et al. [162] reported a patient who had MS presenting with obsessive-compulsive symptoms but he did not comment on the pharmacologic management.

The use of ECT in MS has been reviewed by Hsiao et al. [163] who noted that in 9 cases published, complications were seen in only 1, a patient having catatonia with hemiparesis who developed paraparesis after one ECT. The catatonia improved as did, with time, the paraparetic symptoms. Berrios and Quemada [156] wrote that ECT may be of limited use in MS but no data were cited to support this except for 2 cases wherein neurologic relapse occurred after ECT. There is some evidence that patients with gadolinium-enhancing lesions on MRI are at greater risk for neurological sequellae to ECT [164].

Further pharmacotherapeutic trials assessing the efficacy of various drugs for the myriad neuropsychiatric manifestations of MS are awaited. Pharmacodynamics may possibly be altered in the MS patient, as may be the sensitivity to psychotropics. In order to increase the validity of future studies, attention will have to be paid to controlling for the fluctuating course of the disease in many MS patients.

Stroke

Much work has been done correlating the localization of stroke lesions with specific psychopathology. Patients with major depression and prominent anxiety are more likely to have left cortical lesions. Subcortical lesions are less likely to cause anxiety; symptoms of bipolar mood disorder correlate with right-sided lesions [165]. Depressive symptoms following a stroke are generally severe, longstanding [166] and lead to increased morbidity and mortality. Cushman [167] found that stroke patients with psychiatric comorbidity have greater lengths of stay in hospital and were less frequently discharged to their homes.

Antidepressants have been used in poststroke depression. One double-blind study evaluated the efficacy of nortriptyline in this population [168]. A significantly greater improvement in depression, as measured by the Hamilton and Zung Depression Scales, was found in patients with thromboembolic or hemorrhagic strokes treated with nortriptyline compared to a placebo control group. It must be noted that 6 of 17 patients on active medications dropped out because of side effects; 3 with delirium [168]. Since no particular class of antidepressant has been clearly proven to be superior to others, it is important to consider side effect profiles in choosing an antidepressant. The tendency for MAOIs and cyclic antidepressants to cause orthostasis may prove problematic to patients whose strokes were due to arterial insufficiency. Maprotaline and bupropion lower the seizure threshold and may precipitate convulsions in stroke patients. Fluoxetine, sertaline, and paroxetine are without the α-adrenergic and anticholinergic actions of the cyclic agents, but there has been little published experience with these drugs in poststroke patients. Psychostimulants may be of help in depression secondary to cerebrovascular accidents (CVA).

Trazodone, which has minimumal in vitro anticholinergic activity, was found to improve scores on an activities of daily living scale in poststroke patients with clinical depression, elevated scores on depression scales and/or abnormal dexamethasone suppression tests (DST) [169]. Improvements were not found in nondepressed patients or those treated with placebo. The findings were statistically significant only for patients with nonsuppression on DST.

One retrospective study showed that of 17 patients given the psychostimulants methylphenidate or dextroamphetamine, 82% showed rapid improvement which occurred within 2 days [170]. Kaplitz [171] found that in 44 inpatients diagnosed as 'senile', methylphenidate was superior to placebo in the treatment of withdrawal and apathy [171]. Side effects of the psychostimulants include nausea, tremor, appetite changes and insomnia as well as exacerbation of preexisting anxiety [172].

The one advantage of psychostimulants over other antidepressants is the rapidity of its onset of action. This can produce enough improvement in mood and a subjective increase in well-being to allow patients to tolerate the rigors of rehabilitation. Efficacy beyond the acute stage is unestablished. In Satel and Nelson's [172] review, habituation to the beneficial effects of psychostimulants did not seem to occur in 4 of 5 studies cited. One older study [173] asserted the declining efficacy of stimulants over time.

The use of ECT in poststroke depression has generally been shown to be effective with minimal complications [163, 174]. Death was reported in 2 of 20 patients reported by Shapiro and Goldberg [175], probably in association with significant cardiovascular disease. Murray et al. [174] reviewed the charts of 14 patients treated with ECT poststroke. Twelve of the patients improved and of the 6 patients who had pretreatment cognitive impairment, 5 had improvement in cognition after treatment. Though stroke, per se, is not a contraindication to ECT, one must be sure that enough time has elapsed since the CVA to allow edema to resolve and intracranial pressure to return to normal. Hsiao et al. [163] estimates the risk as minimal when healing has taken place although he offered no exact parameters to assess healing. Four of Murray et al.'s [174] patients received ECT within 1 month of their strokes and there has even been a report of ECT being administered within 4 days of a CVA [176]. Serial imaging studies and neurologic consultation can help determine when it is safe to proceed with convulsive therapy. Prior to administering ECT to a patient with a history of stroke, a search should be made for embolic sources. During treatment, care should be exercized to avoid hyper- or hypotension.

Human Immunodeficiency Virus Spectrum Disorders

Neuropsychiatric manifestations of HIV infection are varied and it is only recently that its CNS effects are being characterized in detail. Histories of patients with AIDS typically include reports of lethargy, withdrawal and other subtle psychiatric manifestations [177]. These may be due to the invasion of CNS tissue by HIV or secondary infections or malignancies. The psychosocial adjustments to the diagnosis itself may produce added symptoms including anxiety and depression [178]. Reports indicate that about 30–40% of AIDS patients have neurologic symptoms at some point in their illnesses [179]. Seemingly unique to AIDS is a syndrome characterized by progressive dementia with motor and behavioral disturbances [180] now termed the AIDS-dementia complex. Kauffman [181] estimates that the AIDS-dementia complex may be the most common neurologic manifestation of AIDS developing in up to 70% of the cases.

It may be useful to categorize symptoms into those that are due to the CNS effects of the HIV infection itself, as well as direct CNS involvement by secondary infections and malignancies versus those that are reactions to the psychosocial implications of the diagnosis. This distinction helps in formulating realistic treatment goals for pharmacotherapy. The current primary treatment for AIDS is zidovudine (AZT). Primary CNS involvement, as exemplified by the AIDS dementia complex, may respond to this treatment. In a study assessing the neuropsychological outcome of AZT treatment in AIDS, it was found that AIDS patients who received AZT showed improved cognition as measured by neuropsychological examination, although affective symptoms were not affected [182]. AZT itself can be quite toxic and may produce neurobehavioral manifestations like psychogenic pain [183], mania [184], coma [185] and other peripheral and central neurologic side effects. Other drugs commonly used in AIDS patients like co-trimoxazole, isoniazid, acyclovir and interferon-α have been associated with neuropsychiatric effects [186]. Where indicated, empirical trials of low doses of high-potency neuroleptics may be done for carefully evaluated target symptoms.

Ostrow writes that patients with HIV infections respond to antidepressants in much the same way as do geriatric patients and that the anticholinergic effects of many of these agents may prove to be problematic [186]. In a chart review, Hintz et al. [187] found that the non-anticholinergic trazodone was better tolerated than several tricyclics and fluoxetine, but was least effective. Imipramine and fluoxetine seemed to have the most favorable balance of adverse reactions and effectiveness. Rabkin and Harrison [188] found that imipramine was effective in 8 of 11 HIV-positive, depressed, gay men, and only caused a transient drop in T4 counts. Of note is that 1 patient who did not respond to imipramine combined with dextroamphetamine improved on fluoxetine.

Psychostimulants may improve mood and cognitive functioning in HIV-infected patients [189, 190]. Use of doses up to 120 mg of methylphenidate [189] and 60 mg of dextroamphetamine [190] have been reported. Some patients who did not respond to methylphenidate improved when switched to dextroamphetamine [190]. Stimulants may be used in combination with other non-MAOI antidepressants, but when used alone have the advantages of lacking α-adrenergic blocking and anticholinergic effects.

Little has been written about the use of the newer antidepressants in HIV-positive patients. As noted above, there have been reports of favorable responses to fluoxetine [187, 188]. The side effect profiles of the newer drugs make them potentially attractive choices in these medically and neurologically compromised patients. In light of the reactions of HIV-positive patients to psychostimulants, the novel antidepressant bupropion may prove to be useful. The epileptogenic properties of bupropion will have to be considered in this at-risk population and there has been a report of bupropion-induced mania in an HIV-positive patient [191]. Finally, ECT can be used to treat depression in patients positive for HIV as long as there is no condition which increases intracranial pressure [192].

For psychotic symptoms, careful trials of low-dose antipsychotics may be instituted. Benzodiazepines may be used for anxiety. Buspirone, a nonsedating, nonbenzodiazepine anxiolytic was reported to cause psychosis in a 52-year-old HIV-positive man [193].

Psychotherapy should always be considered as a treatment option both as adjunctive to medication or as a primary modality especially when the symptoms are clearly secondary to psychosocial adjustment difficulties in the otherwise asymptomatic patient. Keeping this in mind allows for a comprehensive approach to the management of the various neurological and psychiatric manifestations of AIDS.

Central Nervous System Lupus

Systemic lupus erythematosus (SLE) is an autoimmune, inflammatory disease characterized by a chronic course and multiorgan involvement. Neuropsychiatric manifestations are common and include motor deficits, seizures, delirium, psychosis, depression, and phobias [194]. Dementia and autistic behavior have also been documented. Psychiatric manifestations can either precede or occur within 1 year of SLE diagnosis [195]. Work has been done which associates antibodies to ribosomal P proteins with neuropsychiatric manifestations [196] which underscores the immunologic roots of these psychiatric disturbances. Since there have been few studies of the psychopharmacologic management of the psychiatric manifestations of lupus, treatments are emperically based and symptomatically focused. As seizures are a fairly common manifestation of lupus [197, 198], the use of psychotropics may precipitate seizures due to the ability of many psychotropics to lower seizure thresholds. The reader is referred to the section of this paper on seizure disorder for a fuller discussion of this topic. Wong et al. [198] point out that neuropsychiatric symptoms in patients with lupus may be due to concomitant conditions, such as infections. Thus, care must be taken to evaluate lupus patients for all possible causes of mental status changes.

Steroids remain a mainstay in the treatment of lupus and corticosteroids may be helpful in ameliorating neuropsychiatric manifestations of the disease [194]. However, steroids themselves can produce psychosis which seems to be a dose-related phenomenon [199]. Other steroid-related problems include hallucinations, jitteriness, insomnia, depression, and euphoria. However, several groups have reported improvement in symptoms of cerebritis using steroid therapy [200, 201]. Patients with CNS lupus may benefit from plasmapheresis [202].

Among the psychotropics, chlorpromazine has been documented to cause a lupus-like illness with dyspnea, pleural effusions, and elevated antinuclear antibody titer [203]. Perphenazine was implicated in one case of a maculopapular rash, elevated WBC count, and a facial 'butterfly' rash [204]. The symptoms in these lupus-like illnesses tend to be evanescent compared to the 'true' lupus and will often resolve when the offending agent is discontinued.

ECT has been used to treat psychiatric symptoms in patients with SLE. Depression [205], psychosis [205], and catatonia [206, 207] in patient with lupus have responded to ECT. Active cerebritis was clearly present in at least one of the cases presented [207]. There were no reports of neurological sequelae from treatment. ECT may be used in conjunction with aggressive treatment of the lupus [207]. ECT should not be used if there is evidence of increased intracranial pressure.

References

1   Moshkin AV: The permeability of the blood-cerebrospinal fluid barrier in the first 24 hours after cranio-cerebral injury. Laboratornoe Delo 1990;10:47–50.
2   Zhitnukhin I, Sofronov BN: Disordered permeability of the hemato-encephalic barrier in the development of allergic responses to the nervous system. Patolo Ffiziol Exp Ter 1989;5:44–47.
3   Gilman S, Newman SW: Manter and Gatz's Essentials of Clinical Neuroanatomy and Neurophysiology, ed 8. Philadelphia, Davis, 1992.
4   Fenton GW: Psychiatric disorders of epilepsy: Classification and phenomenology; in Reynolds

EH, Trimble MR (eds): Epilepsy and Psychiatry. Edinburgh, Churchill-Livingstone, 1981, pp 12–26.

5 Tedeschi DH, Benigni JP, Elder CJ, Yeager JC, Flanigan JV: Effects of various phenothiazines on minimal electroshock seizure threshold and spontaneous motor activity of mice. J Pharmacol Exp Ther 1958;123:35–38.

6 Chen G, Ensor CR, Bohner B: Studies of drug effects of electrically induced extensor seizures and clinical implications. Arch Int Pharmacodyn 1968;172:183–218.

7 Oliver PA, Luchins DJ, Wyatt RJ: Neuroleptic-induced seizures: An in vitro technique for assessing relative risk. Arch Gen Psychiatry 1982;39:202–209.

8 Itil TM: Effects of psychotropic drugs in qualitatively and quantitatively analyzed human EEG; in Clark WG, del Guidice J (eds): Principles of Psychopharmacology, ed 2. New York, Academic Press, 1978, pp 261–277.

9 Logothetis J: Spontaneous epileptic seizures and electroencephalographic changes in the course of phenothiazine therapy. Neurology 1967;17:869–877.

10 Toone BK, Fenton GW: Epileptic seizures induced by psychotropic drugs. Psychol Med 1977; 7:265–270.

11 Itil TM, Soldatos C: Epileptogenic side effects of psychotropic drugs: Practical recommendations. JAMA 1980;244:1460–1463.

12 Remick RA, Fine SH: Antipsychotic drugs and seizures. J Clin Psychiatry 1979;40:78–80.

13 Devinsky O, Honigfeld G, Patin J: Clozapine-related seizures. Neurology 1991;41:369–371.

14 Mendez MF, Cummings JL, Benson DF: Epilepsy: Psychiatric aspects and use of psychotropics. Psychosomatics 1984;25:883–894.

15 Kaminer Y, Munitz H: Case report: Psychomotor status-like episodes under haloperidol treatment. Br J Psychiatry 1984;145:87–90.

16 Markowitz JC, Brown RP: Seizures with neuroleptics and antidepressants. Gen Hosp Psychiatry 1987;9:135–141.

17 Kiloh LG, Davison K, Osselton JW: An electroencephalographic study of the analeptic effects if imipramine. Electroencephalogr Clin Neurophysiol 1961;13:216–223.

18 Trimble M: Non-monoamine oxidase inhibitor antidepressants and epilepsy: A review. Epilepsia 1978;19:241–250.

19 Lipka LJ, Lathers CM: Psychoactive agents, seizure production, and sudden death in epilepsy. J Clin Pharmacol 1987;27:169–183.

20 Edwards JG: Antidepressants and convulsions. Lancet 1979;ii:1368–1369.

21 Burley DM: A brief note on the problem of epilepsy in antidepressant treatment; in Jukes A (ed): Depression – The Biochemical and Physiologic Role of Ludiomil. Horsham, Ciba, 1977, pp 201–203.

22 Peck AW, Stern WC, Watkinson C: Incidence of seizures during treatment with tricyclic antidepressants drugs and bupropion. J Clin Psychiatry 1983;44(5 sec 2):197–201.

23 Jacob W: Tolerance of trimipramine in general practice. Psychopharmacol Abstr 1964;4:428.

24 Lamont ES: Side effects of pertofran. Br Med J 1965;ii:483.

25 Wedin GP, Oderda GM, Klein-Schwartz W, Gorman RL: Relative toxicity of cyclic antidepressants. Ann Emerg Med 1986;15:797–804.

26 Fromm GH, Amores CY, Thies W: Imipramine in epilepsy. Arch Neurol 1972;27:198–204.

27 Fromm GH, Wessel HB, Glass JD, Alvin JD, Van Horn G: Imipramine in absence and myoclonic-astatic seizures. Neurology 1978;28:953–957.

28 Hurst DL: The use of imipramine in minor motor seizures. Pediatr Neurol 1986;2:13–17.

29 Ojemann LM, Baugh-Bookman C, Dudley DL: Effect of psychotropic medication on seizure control in patients with epilepsy. Neurology 1987;37:1525–1527.

30 Ojemann LM, Friel PN, Trejo WJ, Dudley DL: Effects of doxepin on seizure frequency in depressed epileptic patients. Neurology 1983;33:646–648.

31 Luchins DJ, Oliver AP, Wyatt RJ: Seizures with antidepressants: An in vitro technique to assess relative risk. Epilepsia 1984;25:25–32.

32 Simeon J, Spero M, Fink M: Clinical and EEG studies of doxepin. Psychosomatics 1969;10: 14–17.

33 Preskorn SH, Fast GA: Tricyclic antidepressant-induced seizures and plasma drug concentration. J Clin Psychiatry 1992;53:160–162.

34 Prockop DJ, Shore PA, Brodie BB: Anticonvulsant properties of monoamine oxidase inhibitors. Ann NY Acid Sci 1959;80:643–651.

35 Dessain EC, Schatzberg AF, Woods BT, Cole JO: Maprotaline treatment in depression: A perspective on seizures. Arch Gen Psychiatry 1986;43:86–90.

36 Horne RL, Ferguson JM, Pope HG, Hudson JI, Lineberry CG, Ascher J, Cato A: Treatment of bulimia with bupropion: A multicenter controlled trial. J Clin Psychiatry 1988;49:262–266.

37 Johnston JA, Lineberry CG, Ascher JA, Davidson J, Khayrallah MA, Feighner JP, Stark P: A 102-center prospective study of seizure in association with bupropion. J Clin Psychiatry 1991;52:450–456.

38 Davidson J: Seizures and bupropion: A review. J Clin Psychiatry 1989;50:256–261.

39 Goldberg JP: Bupropion dose, seizures, women, and age. J Clin Psychiatry 1990;51:388–389.

40 Litovitz TL, Troutman WG. Amoxapine overdose: Seizures and fatalities. JAMA 1983;250:1069–1071.

41 Goldberg MJ, Spector R: Amoxapine overdose: Report of two patients with severe neurologic damage. Ann Intern Med 1982;96:463–464.

42 Bowdan ND: Seizure possibly caused by trazodone HCL. Am J Psychiatry 1983;140:642.

43 Lefkowitz D, Kilgo G, Lee S: Seizures and trazodone therapy. Arch Gen Psychiatry 1985;42:523.

44 Tasini M: Complex partial seizures in a patient receiving trazodone. J Clin Psychiatry 1986;47:318–319.

45 Ware MR, Stewart RB: Seizure associated with fluoxetine therapy. DICP 1989;23:428.

46 Wernicke JF: The side effect profile and safety of fluoxetine. J Clin Psychiatry 1985;46(3 sec 2):59–67.

47 Cooper GL: The safety of fluoxetine: An update. Br J Psychiatry 1988;153(suppl 3):77–86.

48 Sacristan JA, Iglesias C, Arellano F, Lequerica J: Absence seizures induced by lithium: Possible interaction with fluoxetine. Am J Psychiatry 1991;148:146–147.

49 Grady TA, Pigott TA, L'Heureux F, Murphy DL: Seizure associated with fluoxetine and adjuvant buspirone therapy. J Clin Psychopharmacol 1992;12:70–71.

50 Hargrave R, Martinez D, Bernstein AJ: Fluoxetine-induced seizures. Psychosomatics 1992;33:236–237.

51 Pasini A, Tortorella A, Gale K: Anticonvulsant effect of intranigral fluoxetine. Brain Res 1992;593:287–290.

52 Prendiville S, Gale K: Anticonvulsant effect of fluoxetine on focally evoked limbic motor seizures in rats. Epilepsia 1993;34:381–384.

53 Wroblewski BA, Leary JM, Phelan AM, Whyte J, Manning K: Methylphenidate and seizure frequency in brain injured patients with seizure disorder. J Clin Psychiatry 1992;53:86–89.

54 Physicians' Desk Reference, ed 46. Montvale, Medical Economics Data, 1992.

55 Livingston S, Pauli L: Dextroamphetamine for epilepsy. JAMA 1975;223:278–279.

56 Appleby JG: Use of dextroamphetamine for epilepsy. JAMA 1975:233:278–279.

57 Feldman H, Crumrine P, Handen BL, Alvin R, Tedori J: Methylphenidate in children with seizures and attention deficit disorder. Am J Dis Child 1989;143:1081–1086.

58 Rosenstein DL, Nelson JC, Jacobs SC: Seizures associated with antidepressants: a review. J Clin Psychiatry 1993;54:289–299.

59 Sackheim HA, Decina P, Prohovnik I, Malitz S, Resor SR: Anticonvulsant and antidepressant properties of electroconvulsive therapy: A proposed mechanism of action. Biol Psychiatry 1983;18:1301–1310.

60 Abrams R: Electroconvulsive Therapy, ed 2. New York, Oxford University Press, 1992.

61 Blackwood DH, Cull RE, Freeman CPL, Evans JI, Mawdsley C: A study of the incidence of epilepsy following ECT. J Neurol Neurosurg Psychiatry 1980;43:1098–1102.

62 Jefferson JW, Greist JH, Ackerman DL, Carroll JA: Lithium Encyclopedia for Clinical Practice, ed 2. Washington, American Psychiatric Press, 1987, pp 463–463.

63 Minabe Y, Emori K, Kurachi M: Effects of chronic lithium treatment on limbic seizure generation in the cat. Psychopharmacology (Berlin) 1988;96:391–394.

64 Meyers BS, Kalayam B: Update in Geriatric Psychopharmacology. Adv Psychosomatic Med 1989;19:114–137.

65 Whalley LJ, Bradnock J: Treatment of the classical manifestations of dementia and confusion. Br Med Bull 1990;1:169–180.

66 Baldessarini RJ: Chemotherapy in Psychiatry: Principles and Practice (rev). Cambridge, Harvard University Press, 1985.

67 Altman H, Mehta D, Evenson RC, Sletter IW: Behavioral effects of drug therapy on psychogeriatric inpatients. I. Chlorpromazine and thioridazine. J Am Geriatr Soc 1973;21:241–248.

68 Butler FR, Burgio LD, Engel BT: Neuroleptics and behaviour: A comparative study. J Gerontol Nurs 1987;13:15–19.

69 Sugerman A, William BH, Adlerstein A: Haloperidol in the psychiatric disorders of old age. Am J Psychiatry 1964;120:1190–1192.

70 Rada RT, Kellner R: Thiothixene in the treatment of geriatric patients with chronic organic brain syndrome. J Am Geriatr Soc 1976;24:105–107.

71 Petrie WM, Bar TA, Berney S, Fujimori, Guy W, Ragheb GM, Wilson WH, Schaffer JD: Loxapine in psychogeriatrics: A placebo and standard-controlled clinical investigation. J Clin Psychopharmacol 1982;2:122.

72 Bohon RJ, Gershon S: Antipsychotics in the elderly. Acta Psychiatr Scand 1990;82(suppl 358): 170–175.

73 Gershon S, Eison MA: The ideal anxiolytic. Psychiatr Ann 1987;17:156–170.

74 Petursson H, Lader MH: Benzodiazepine dependence. Br J Addict 1981;76:133–145.

75 Greendyke RM, Kanter DR: Therapeutic effects of pindolol on behavioral disturbances associated with organic brain disease: A double blind study. J Clin Psychiatry 1986;47:423–426.

76 Yudofsky S: Propranolol in the treatment of rage and violent behavior in patients with chronic brain syndromes. Am J Psychiatry 1981;138:218–230.

77 Simpson DM, Foster D: Improvement in organically disturbed behavior with trazodone treatment. J Clin Psychiatry 1986;47:191–193.

78 Fava GA, Sonino N, Wise TN: Management of depression in medical patients. Psychother Psychosom 1988;49:81–102.

79 Hollister LE: Drugs for mental disorder of old age. JAMA 1978; 234:195–198.

80 Kaufman MA, Murray GB, Cassem NH: Use of psychostimulants in medically ill depressed patients. Psychosomatics 1982;23:817–819.

81 Fisch RZ: Methylphenidate for medical inpatients. Int J Psychiatry Med 1985/1986;15:75–79.

82 Mallory FW, Small IF, Miller MJ, Milstein V; Stout JR: Changes in neuropsychological test performance after electroconvulsive therapy. Biol Psychiatry 1982;17:61–67.

83 Frith CD, Stevens M, Johnstone EC, Deakin JFW, Lawler P, Crow TJ: Effects of ECT and depression on various aspects of memory. Br J Psychiatry 1983;142:610–617.

84 Dubovsky SL: Use of electroconvulsive therapy for patients with neurological disease. Hosp Community Psychiatry 1986;37:819–825.

85 Harvey NS: Psychiatric disorders in parkinsonism. 1. Functional illness and personality. Psychosomatics 1986;27:91–102.

86 Cummings JL: Depression and Parkinson's disease: A review. Am J Psychiatry 1992;149: 443–454.

87 Huber SJ, Paulson GW, Shuttleworth EC: Relationship of motor symptoms, intellectual impairment, and depression in Parkinson's disease. J Neurol Neurosurg Psychiatry 1988;51:855–858.

88 Robins AH: Depression in patients with parkinsonism. Br J Psychiatry 1976;128:141–145.

89 Ehmann TS, Beninger JR, Gawel MJ, Riopelle RJ: Depressive symptoms in Parkinson's disease: A comparison with disabled control subjects. J Geriatr Psychiatry Neurol 1990;2:3–9.

90 Marsh GG, Markham CH: Does levodopa alter depression and psychopathology in parkinsonism patients? J Neurol Neurosurg Psychiatry 1973;36:925–935.

91 Damasio AR, Lobo-Antunes J, Macedo C: Psychiatric aspects in parkinsonism treated with *l*-dopa. J Neurol Neurosurg Psychiatry 1971;34:502–507.

92   Jouvent R, Abensour P, Bonner AM, Widlocher D, Agid Y, Lhermitte F: Antiparkinsonian and antidepressant effects of high doses of bromocriptine: A independent comparison. J Affective Disord 1983;5:141–145.

93   Youdim MBH, Finberg JPM, Wajsbort J: Monoamine oxidase type B inhibitors in the treatment of Parkinson's disease. Prog Med Chem 1984;21:137–167.

94   Tetrud JW, Langston JW: The effect of deprenyl (selegiline) on the natural history of Parkinson's disease. Science 1989;245:519–522.

95   Koller WC, Giron LT: Selegiline HCl: selective MAO-type B inhibitor. Neurology 1990;40 (suppl 3):58–60.

96   Strang RR: Imipramine in treatment of parkinsonism: A double-blind placebo study. Br Med J 1965;ii:33–34.

97   Laitinen L: Desipramine in treatment of Parkinson's disease. Acta Neurol Scand 1969;45: 109–113.

98   Andersen J, Aabro E, Gulmann N, Hjelmsted A, Pedersen HE: Anti-depressive treatment in Parkinson's disease: A controlled trial of the effect of nortriptyline in patients with Parkinson's disease treated with *l*-dopa. Acta Neurol Scand 1980;62:210–219.

99   Driver PS: Depression treatment in Parkinson's disease. DICP 1991;25:137–138.

100   Bedard P, Parkes JD, Marsden CD: Nomifensine in Parkinson's disease. Br J Clin Pharmacol 1977;4(suppl):187–190.

101   Park DM, Findley LJ, Teychenne PF: Nomifensin in parkinsonism. Br J Clin Pharmacol 1977; 4(suppl):185–186.

102   Park DM, Findley LJ, Hanks G, Sandler M: Nomifensine: Effect in parkinsonian patients not receiving levodopa. J Neurol Neurosurg 1981;44:352–354.

103   Goetz CG, Tanner CM, Klawans HL: Bupropion in Parkinson's disease. Neurology 1984;34: 1092–1094.

104   Liberzon I, Dequardo JR, Silk KR: Bupropion and delirium. Am J Psychiatry 1990;147: 1689–1690.

105   Parkes JD, Tarsy D, Marsden CD, Bovill KT, Phipps JA, Rose P, Asselman P: Amphetamines in the treatment of Parkinson's disease. J Neurol Neurosurg Psychiat 1975;38:232–237.

106   Cantello R, Aguggia M, Gilli M, Delsedime M, Ciardo Cutin I, Riccio A, Mutani R: Major depression in Parkinson's disease and the mood response to intravenous methylphenidate: Possible role of the 'hedonic' dopamine synapse. J Neurol Neurosurg Psychiatry 1989;52:724–731.

107   Caley CF, Friedman JH: Does fluoxetine exacerbate Parkinson's disease? J Clin Psychiatry 1992;53:278–282.

108   Suchowersky O, deVries J: Possible interactions between deprenyl and Prozac. Can J Neurol Sci 1990;17:352–353.

109   Montastruc JL, Chamontin B, Senard JM, Tran MA, Rascol O, Llau ME, Rascol A: Pseudophaeochromocytoma in a parkinsonian patient treated with fluoxetine plus selegiline. Lancet 1993;341:555.

110   Steur ENHJ: Increase in parkinson disability after fluoxetine medication. Neurology 1993;43: 211–213.

111   Greenberg R, Meyers BS: Treatment of major depression and parkinson's disease with combined phenelzine and amantadine. Am J Psychiatry 1985;142:273–274.

112   Bartholini G, Scatton B, Zivkovic B, Lloyd KG: GABA receptor agonists and extrapyramidal motor function: Therapeutic implications for Parkinson's disease. Adv Neurol 1987;45:79–83.

113   Ludwig CL, Weinberger DR, Bruno G, Gillespie M, Bakker K, LeWitt PA, Chase TN: Buspirone, Parkinson's disease, and the locus ceruleus. Clin Neuropharmacol 1986;4:373–378.

114   Lebensohn ZM, Jenkins RB: Improvement of parkinsonism in depressed patients treated with ECT. Am J Psychiatry 1975;132:283–285.

115   Atre-Vaidya N, Jambala VC: Electroconvulsive therapy in parkinsonism with affective disorder. Br J Psychiatry 1988;152:55–58.

116   Douyon R, Serby M, Klutchko B, Rotrosen J: ECT and Parkinson's disease: A 'naturalistic'-study. Am J Psychiatry 1989;146:1451–1455.

117   Holcomb HH, Sternberg DE, Heninger GR: Effects of electroconvulsive therapy on mood,

parkinsonism and tardive dyskinesia in a depressed patient: ECT and dopamine systems. Biol Psychiatry 1983;18:865–873.

118 Young RC, Alexopoulos GS, Shamoian CA: Dissociation of motor response from mood and cognition in a parkinsonian patient treated with ECT. Biol Psychiatry 1985;20:566–569.

119 Hurwitz TA, Calne DB, Waterman K: Treatment of dopaminomimetic psychosis in Parkinson's disease with electroconvulsive therapy. Can J Neurol Sci 1988;15:32–34.

120 Balldin J, Granerus AK, Lindstedt G, Modigh K, Walinder J: Predictors for improvement after electroconvulsive therapy in parkinsonian patients with on-off symptoms. J Neural Transm 1981;52:199–211.

121 Andersen K, Balldin J, Gottfries CG, Granerus A-K, Modigh K, Svennerholm L, Wallin A: A double-blind evaluation of electroconvulsive therapy in Parkinson's disease with 'on-off' phenomena. Acta Neurol Scand 1987;76:191–199.

122 Ward C, Stern GM, Pratt RTC, McKenna P: Electroconvulsive therapy in parkinsonian patients with the 'on-off' syndrome. J Neural Transm 1980;49:133–135.

123 Oh JJ, Rummans TA, O'Connor MK, Ahlskog JE: Cognitive impairment after ECT in patients with Parkinson's disease and psychiatric illness. Am J Psychiatry 1992;149:271.

124 Zervas IM, Fink M: ECT and delirium in Parkinson's disease. Am J Psychiatry 1992;149:1758.

125 Harsch HH, Miller M, Young LD: Induction of mania by *l*-dopa in a nonbipolar patient. J Clin Psychopharmacol 1985;5:338–339.

126 Coffey CE, Ross DR, Ferren EL, Sullivan JL, Olanow CW: Treatment of the 'on-off' phenomenon in parkinsonism with lithium carbonate. Ann Neurol 1982;12:375–379.

127 Harvey NS: Psychiatric disorders in parkinsonism. 2. Organic cerebral states and drug reactions. Psychosomatics 1986;27:175–185.

128 Hale MS, Bellizzi J: Low dose perphenazine and levodopa/carbidopa therapy in a patient with parkinsonism and a psychotic illness. J Nerv Ment Dis 1980;168:312–314.

129 Baldessarini RJ, Frankenburg FR: Drug therapy: Clozapine: A novel antipsychotic agent. N Engl J Med 1991;324:746–754.

130 Friedman JH, Lannon MC: Clozapine in the treatment of psychosis in Parkinson's disease: Neurology 1989;39:1219–1221.

131 Kahn N, Freeman A, Juncos JL, Manning D, Watts RL: Clozapine is beneficial for psychosis in Parkinson's disease. Neurology 1991;41:1699–1700.

132 Pfeiffer RF, Kang J, Graber B, Hofman R, Wilson J: Clozapine for psychosis in Parkinson's disease. Mov Disord 1990;5:239–242.

133 Whitehouse PJ, Friedland RP, Strauss ME: Neuropsychiatric aspects of degenerative dementias associated with motor dysfunction; in Yudofsky SC, Hales RE (eds): The American Psychiatric Press Textbook of Neuropsychiatry, ed 2. Washington, American Psychiatric Press, 1992, pp 585–604.

134 Byers RK, Gilles FH, Fung C: Huntington's disease in children: Neuropathologic study in four cases. Neurology 1973;23:561–569.

135 Myers RH, Sax DS, Koroshetz WJ, Mastromauro C, Cupples LA, Kiely DK, Pettengill FJ, Bird ED: Factors associated with slow progression in Huntington's disease. Arch Neurol 1991; 48:800–804.

136 Gusella JF, Wexler NS, Conneally PM, Naylor SL, Anderson MA, Tanzi RE, Watkins PC, Ottina K, Wallace MR, Sakaguchi AY, Young AB, Shoulson I, Bonilla E, Martin JB: A polymorphic DNA marker genetically linked to Huntington's disease. Nature 1983;306:234–238.

137 Folstein SE, Abbot MH, Chase GA, Jensen BA, Folstein MF: The association of affective disorder with Huntington's disease in a case series and in families. Psychol Med 1983;13:537–542.

138 Caine ED, Shoulson I: Psychiatric syndromes in Huntington's disease. Am J Psychiatry 1983; 140:728–733.

139 Klawans HL: Chorea. Can J Neurol Sci 1987;14:536–540.

140 Shoulson I: Huntington's disease: Functional capacities in patients treated with neuroleptic and antidepressant drugs. Neurology 1981;31:1333–1335.

141 Moss JH, Stewart DE: Iatrogenic parkinsonism in Huntington's chorea. Can J Psychiatry 1986; 31:865–866.

142 Schott K, Ried S, Stevens I, Dichgans J: Neuroleptically induced dystonia in Huntington's disease: A case report. Eur Neurol 1989;29:39–40.

143 Sajatovic M, Verbanac P, Ramirez LF, Meltzer HY: Clozapine treatment of psychiatric symptoms resistant to neuroleptic treatment in patients with Huntington's chorea. Neurology 1991;41:156.

144 Stewart JT: Huntington's disease. Am Fam Physician 1988;37:105–114.

145 Ford MF: Treatment of depression in Huntington's disease with monoamine oxidase inhibitors. Br J Psychiatry 1986;149:654–656.

146 Stewart JT, Mounts ML, Clark RL: Aggressive behavior in Huntington's disease: Treatment with propranolol. J Clin Psychiatry 1987;48:106–108.

147 Stewart JT: Paradoxical aggressive effect of propranolol in a patient with Huntington's disease. J Clin Psychiatry 1987;48:385–386.

148 von Haften AH, Jensen CF: Paradoxical response to pindolol treatment for aggression in a patient with Huntington's disease. J Clin Psychiatry 1989;50:230–231.

149 Leonard DP, Kidson MA, Shannon PJ, Brown J: Double-blind trial of lithium carbonate and haloperidol in Huntington's chorea. Lancet 1974;ii:1208–1209.

150 Caraceni T, Giovannini P, Girotti F, Avanzini G: Pharmacology of Huntington's chorea: Personal experience. Eur Neurol 1977;16:42–50.

151 Petersen RC, Kokmen E: Cognitive and psychiatric abnormalities in multiple sclerosis. Mayo Clin Proc 1989;64:657–663.

152 Skegg K, Corwin PA, Skegg DC: How often is multiple sclerosis mistaken for a psychiatric disorder? Psychol Med 1988;18:733–736.

153 Ontiveros A, Fontaine R: Panic attacks and multiple sclerosis. Biol Psychiatry 1990;27:672–673.

154 Rudick RA, Schiffer RB, Herndon RM: Drug treatment of multiple sclerosis. Semin Neurol 1987;7:150–159.

155 Minden SL, Schiffer RB: Depression and mood disorders in multiple sclerosis. Neuropsychiatry Neuropsychol Behav Neurol 1991;4:62–77.

156 Berrios GE, Quemada JI: Depressive illness in multiple sclerosis. Clinical and theoretical aspects of the association. Br J Psychiatry 1990;156:10–16.

157 Schiffer RB, Wineman NM: Antidepressant pharmacotherapy of depression associated with multiple sclerosis. Am J Psychiatry 1990;147:1493–1497.

158 Flax JW, Gray J, Herbert J: Effect of fluoxetine on patients with multiple sclerosis. Am J Psychiatry 1991;148:1603.

159 Browning WN: Exacerbation of symptoms of multiple sclerosis in a patient taking fluoxetine. Am J Psychiatry 1990;147:1089.

160 Schiffer RB, Herndon RM, Rudick RA: Treatment of pathological laughing and weeping with amitriptyline. N Engl J Med 1985;312:1480–1482.

161 Ron MA, Logsdail SJ: Psychiatric morbidity in multiple sclerosis: A clinical and MRI study. Psychol Med 1989;19:887–895.

162 George MS, Kellner CH, Fossey MD: Obsessive-compulsive symptoms in a patient with multiple sclerosis. J Nerv Ment Dis 1989;177:304–305.

163 Hsiao JK, Messenheimer JA, Evans DL: ECT in neurological disorders. Convuls Ther 1987;3: 121–136.

164 Mattingly G, Baker K, Zorumski CF, Figiel GS: Multiple sclerosis and ECT: Possible value of gadolinium-enhanced magnetic resonance scans for identifying high-risk patients. J Neuropsychiatry Clin Neurosci 1992;4:145–151.

165 Robinson RG, Starkstein SE: Current research in affective disorders following stroke. J Neuropsychiatry Clin Neurosci 1990;2:1–14.

166 Messner M, Messner E: Mood disorder following stroke. Compr Psychiatry 1988;29:22–27.

167 Cushman LA: Secondary neuropsychiatric complications in stroke: Implications for acute care. Arch Phys Med Rehabil 1988;69:877–879.

168 Lipsey JR, Robinson RG, Pearlson GD, Rao K, Price TR: Nortriptyline treatment for poststroke depression: A double-blind trial. Lancet 1984;i:297–300.

169 Reding MJ, Orto LA, Winter SW, Fortuna IM, DiPonte P, McDowell FH: Antidepressant therapy after stroke: A double-blind trial. Arch Neurol 1986;43:763–765.

170 Masand P, Pickett P, Murray GB: Psychostimulants for secondary depression in medical illness. Psychosomatics 1991;32:203–208.

171 Kaplitz S: Withdrawn, apathetic geriatric patients responsive to methylphenidate. J Am Geriatr Soc 1975;23:271–276.

172 Satel SL, Nelson JC: Stimulants in the treatment of depression: A critical overview. J Clin Psychiatry 1989;50:241–249.

173 Wilbur DL, MacLean AR, Allen EV: Clinical observations on the effect of benzadrine sulfate. JAMA 1937;109:549–554.

174 Murray GB, Shea V, Conn DK: Electroconvulsive therapy for post-stroke depression. J Clin Psychiatry 1986;47:258–260.

175 Shapiro MF, Goldberg HH: Electroconvulsive therapy in patients with structural disease of the central nervous system. Am J Med Sci 1957;233:186–195.

176 Alexopoulos GS, Shamoian CJ, Lucas J, Weisner N, Berger H: Medical problems of geriatric patients and younger controls during electroconvulsive therapy. J Am Geriatr Soc 1984;32:651–654.

177 Perry S, Jacobsen P: Neuropsychiatric manifestations of AIDS-spectrum disorders. Hosp Community Psychiatry 1986;37:135–142.

178 Fullilove MT: Anxiety and stigmatizing aspects of HIV infection. J Clin Psychiatry 1989; 50(11 suppl):5–8.

179 Detmer WM, Lu FG: Neuropsychiatric complications of AIDS: A literature review. Int Psychiatry Med 1986–7;16:21–29.

180 Navia BA, Jordan BD, Price RW: The AIDS dementia complex. I. Clinical features. Ann Neurol 1986;19:517–524.

181 Kaufman DM: Clinical Neurology for Psychiatrists, ed 3. Philadelphia, Saunders, 1986, pp 127–131.

182 Schmitt FA, Bigley JW, McKinnis R, Logue PE, Evans RW, Drucker JL, the AZT Collaborative Working Group: Neuropsychological outcome of zidovudine (AZT) treatment of patients with AIDS and AIDS-related complex. N Engl J Med 1988;319:1573–1578.

183 Levitt AJ, Lippert GP: Psychogenic panic after zidovudine therapy: The therapeutic benefit of an N of 1 trial. Can Med Assoc J 1990;142:341–2.

184 Wright JM, Sachdev PS, Perkins RJ, Rodriquez P: Zidovudine-related mania. Med J Aust 1989;150:339–41.

185 Riedel RR, Clarenbach P, Reetz KP: Coma during azidothymidine therapy for AIDS. J Neurol 1989;236:185.

186 Ostrow P, Grant F, Atkinson H: Assessment and management of the AIDS patient with neuropsychiatric disturbances. J Clin Psychiatry 1988;49(5 suppl):14–22.

187 Hintz S, Kuck J, Peterkin JJ, Volk DM, Zisook S: Depression in the context of human immunodificiency virus infection: Implications for treatment. J Clin Psychiatry 1990;51:497–501.

188 Rabkin JG, Harrison WM: Effect of imipramine on depression and immune status in a sample of men with HIV infection. Am J Psychiatry 1990;147:495–497.

189 Fernandez F, Levy JK, Galizzi H: Response of HIV-related depression to psychostimulants: Case reports. Hosp Community Psychiatry 1988;39:628–631.

190 Holmes VF, Fernandez F, Levy JK: Psychostimulant response in AIDS-related complex patients. J Clin Psychiatry 1989;50:5–8.

191 Fichtner CG: Bupropion-associated mania in a patient with HIV infection. J Clin Psychopharmacol 1992;12:366–367.

192 Schaerf FW, Miller RR, Lipsey JR, McPherson RW: ECT for major depression in four patients infected with human immunodeficiency virus. Am J Psychiatry 1989;146:782–784.

193 Trachman SB: Buspirone-induced psychosis in a human immunodeficiency virus-infected man. Psychosomatics 1992;33:332–335.

194 Adelman DC, Saltiel E; Klinenberg JR: The neuropsychiatric manifestations of systemic lupus erythematosis: An overview. Semin Arthritis Rheum 1986;15:185–199.

195 Feinglass EJ, Arnett FC, Dorsch CA, Zizic TM, Stevens MB: Neuropsychiatric manifestations of systemic lupus erythematosis: Diagnosis, clinical spectrum, and the relationship to other features of the disease. Medicine 1976;55:323–339.

196 Scheebaum AB, Singleton JD, West SG, Blodgett JK, Allen LG, Cheronis JC, Kotzin BC: Association of psychiatric manifestations with antibodies to ribosomal P proteins in systemic lupus erythematosis. Am J Med 1991;90:54–62.
197 Buchbinder R, Littlejohn GO, Hall S, Ryan PF: Neuropsychiatric manifestations of systemic lupus erythematosis. Aust NZ J Med 1988;18:679–684.
198 Wong KL, Woo EKW, Yu YL, Wong RWS: Neurological manifestations of systemic lupus erythematosis: A prospective study. Q J Med 1991;81:857–870.
199 The Boston Collaborative Drug Surveillance Program: Acute adverse reactions to prednisone in relation to dosage. Clin Pharmacol Ther 1972;13:694–698.
200 Fessel WJ: Megadose corticosteroid therapy in systemic lupus erythematosis. J Rheumatol 1980;7:486–500.
201 Isenberg DA, Morrow MJW, Snaith ML: Methylprednisolone pulse therapy in the treatment of systemic lupus erythematosis. Ann Rheum Dis 1982;41:347–351.
202 Fruchter L, Gauthier B, Marino F: The use of plasmapheresis in a patient with systemic lupus erythematosis and necrotizing cutaneous ulcers. J Rheumatol 1983;10:341–343.
203 Goldman LS, Hudson JI, Weddington WW: Lupus-like illness associated with chlorpromazine. Am J Psychiatry 1980;137:1613–1614.
204 Gold MS, Sweeney DR: Perphenazine-induced systemic lupus erythematosis-like syndrome. J Nerv Ment Dis 1978;166:442–445.
205 Allen RE, Pitts FN: ECT for depressed patients with lupus erythematosis. Am J Psychiatry 1978;135:367–368.
206 Mac DS, Pardo MP: Systemic lupus erythematosis and catatonia: A case report. J Clin Psychiatry 1983;44:155–156.
207 Fricchione GL, Kaufman LD, Gruber BC, Fink M: Electroconvulsive therapy and cyclophosphamide in combination for severe neuropsychiatric lupus with catatonia. Am J Med 1990; 88:442–443.

Paul A. Silver, MD, Department of Psychiatry, Georgetown University Medical Center, 3800 Reservoir Road, NW, Washington, DC 20007 (USA)

Silver PA (ed): Psychotropic Drug Use in the Medically Ill.
Adv Psychosom Med. Basel, Karger, 1994, vol 21, pp 90–106

Psychotropic Medications and the Skin

Lois E. Krahn[a], Richard L. Goldberg[b]

[a] Department of Psychiatry and Psychology, Mayo Clinic and Foundation,
   Rochester, Minn., and
[b] Department of Psychiatry, Georgetown University Medical Center,
   Washington, D. C., USA

The relationship between psychotropic medications and the skin is multi-faceted and, accordingly, relevant to practitioners who treat either psychiatric or dermatologic disorders. This chapter reviews this complex relationship by focusing on three general areas. The cutaneous side effects of many commonly used psychotropic medications; the expanding use of psychotropic medications for the treatment of dermatologic disorders; and two psychiatric disorders with cutaneous manifestations – trichotillomania and delusions of parasitosis.

Cutaneous Side Effects of Psychotropic Medications

Lithium

A great deal has been written about the association between lithium and psoriasis [1–8]. Several studies and case reports describe patients with pre-existing psoriasis whose skin disease worsened after the initiation of lithium and occasionally even became resistant to previously effective therapies. Nonetheless, the nature of the relationship between lithium and psoriasis remains unclear. Not all patients with psoriasis are adversely affected by lithium and having the condition is not considered a contraindication to lithium therapy [1]. However, potentially lethal reactions may be seen as reported by Pande et al. [2]. Lithium was associated with the development of generalized pustular psoriasis, a potentially life-threatening disease, in 1 patient previously diagnosed with stable plaque-type psoriasis. However, causality was difficult to establish because the patient discontinued the treatment of her psoriasis with methotrexate when she became manic. There are also a few reports of patients who developed psoriasis de novo after initiation of lithium therapy [5, 10, 11, 14]. The incidence is unknown but thought to be small. In some cases, these patients have had a family history of the disease but in other instances, psoriasis has been precipitated in patients with no prior personal or family history [3].

The time of onset of lithium-induced psoriasis ranges from a number of weeks to years after the initiation of lithium. The inability of investigators to delineate a clear temporal relationship between inauguration of lithium therapy and the development or worsening of psoriasis may be due to the variability in the natural onset of the disease [4]. Generally, it takes longer for lithium to precipitate psoriasis de novo than to worsen a pre-existing case. Usually, the psoriasis improves when lithium is discontinued; however, in at least one reported case, psoriasis continued to be unimproved after lithium was stopped [5]. There are only a few reports of patients with lithium-associated psoriasis being rechallenged and these provocative tests tend to be positive [1, 3, 4]. Lithium can induce or worsen psoriasis even at a therapeutic level. Lithium-associated psoriasis is often more resistant to conventional treatment, especially in patients with de novo psoriasis [6]. In some cases, dose reduction can be helpful, but at other times lithium discontinuation is indicated [1, 4, 6].

A proposed mechanism for lithium's effect on psoriasis involves its inhibitory action on the adenocyclase/cyclic AMP system in psoriatic plaques. A decrease in cyclic AMP is thought to directly influence epithelial cell proliferation and increase the mobility and phagocytic activity of polymorphonuclear leukocytes [7, 8]. Lithium may also trigger changes in keratinocyte regulation [1].

Acne is another skin disorder associated with lithium therapy. The actual incidence is unknown, but many investigators presume that the problem is relatively common. Numerous cases of de novo acne and acneiform reactions have been reported as well as the exacerbation of preexisting acne [9, 11, 12, 14]. One retrospective study comparing 91 lithium-treated patients with a control group of 44 patients treated with other medications found that 5% of the men and 15% of the women on lithium developed acneiform conditions as opposed to 6 and 4% of the male und female controls, respectively [5].

Lithium-induced acne can be distinguished from acne vulgaris because it typically develops on the forearms and legs rather than the face. The pustules tend to be uniform and at the same stage of development. Also comedones and cysts are usually not present in lithium-induced acne [9]. The onset or exacerbation of acne often occurs shortly after lithium is initiated and with the lithium levels in the normal range [10]. Some authors, however, warn that the sudden onset or worsening of acne may indicate that the lithium level is elevated. This latter view may be true since lithium-induced acne appears to be more dose dependent than any other dermatological side effect [9]. Susceptible patients develop acne when restarted on lithium [11].

Acne tends to clear quickly once lithium is discontinued, but withdrawing lithium is not always necessary to treat acneiform reactions. For example, one report demonstrated that lithium-induced acne was successfully treated with tretinoin, a topical form of retinoic acid, in combination with tetracycline [12]. It is important, though, to consider that tretinoin is related to isotretoin which has multiple side effects including teratogenicity, hypertriglyceridemia, cheilitis and conjunctivitis. Also, tetracycline must be used with caution in treating lithium-induced acneiform eruptions because sustained release lithium and tetracycline can interact to result in renal insufficiency and resultant toxic lithium levels [13]. In most cases though, acne secondary to lithium treatment is difficult to treat with standard therapeutic regimes. One case report described a woman with an acneiform rash on her face, including cheilosis at the corners of her mouth, who was treated with systemic tetracycline and then monocycline along with a topical compound of lincomycin and hydrocortisone without response. Her acne improved only after discontinuation of the lithium [14].

Like psoriasis, lithium-associated acne is believed to be related to decreased cyclic AMP activity. More specifically, acne may develop because decreased cyclic AMP activity induces lysosomal release from leukocytes and also leads to prolonged neutrophil survival [9].

Lithium has also been linked with folliculitis. One study described 12 patients with hyperkeratotic, erythematous, follicular papules on their extremities. These asymptomic lesions appeared 1–12 months after lithium was initiated. The course of the folliculitis can differ significantly: in 3 patients the symptoms cleared when lithium was discontinued (1 patient had a positive and then subsequently negative lithium rechallenge); in 6 patients, the condition cleared without discontinuing lithium, and in 2 patients a topical steroid cream was tried with only one person showing a modest response. The authors concluded that folliculitis does not warrant discontinuing lithium [15].

Alopecia has been reported as a rare side effect of lithium [16–23]. In evaluating alopecia associated with lithium, it is essential to rule out lithium-induced hypothyroidism as the cause of hair loss. A relationship between lithium and alopecia is strongly suggested by numerous case reports, but the nature of the alopecia is difficult to characterize due to the variety of presentations reported [16–23]. In general, scalp hair is affected more than body hair by lithium. Dawber reported 7 patients who initially experienced mild hair loss that progressed to diffuse alopecia. These patients were all continued on lithium despite this side effect and none developed total baldness [16]. Other reports have described one patient who developed alopecia totalis after 2 months of lithium treatment as well as one whose hair loss progressed to alopecia universalis [17, 18].

A Scottish study attempted to determine the incidence of lithium-associated hair loss and found that of 99 patients, 17% had hair thinning and 23% stated their hair lost its curl after lithium treatment was initiated [19]. Yassa [20] surveyed 50 patients, 26 female and 24 male, and found an incidence of 11.5% scalp hair loss in women and none in men. All of the affected patients had been on lithium for at least 5 years and the alopecia was noted to have an abrupt onset, a duration of 6 months to 1 year and spontaneous resolution. Overall, these studies indicate that the majority of affected patients tend to be female. The onset of alopecia varies from several months to over ten years after the initiation of lithium therapy [21]. In most cases lithium can be continued despite alopecia since the hair loss often cases spontaneously and rarely progresses to total baldness [16, 17, 22, 23].

The mechanism for lithium-associated hair loss remains unknown although lithium is known to accumulate in the hair of patients to whom it is prescribed. However, higher concentrations have not been found in the hair of patients with alopecia [22]. Whether lithium exerts a direct toxic effect on hair follicles or causes hair loss by inducing subclinical hypothyroidism is unclear. Additionally, the role of emotional stress in hair loss represents a confounding factor in establishing a clear causal relationship between lithium and alopecia.

A large variety of other skin disorders have also been associated with lithium therapy. There are several reports of pruritic maculopapular rashes. Callaway et al. [24] reported on a series of 5 patients who had dermatologic side effects, including 4 with pruritic maculopapular rashes (2 of whom also had associated cutaneous ulcers of the anterior tibial region). The 5th patient developed an ulcer without an associated rash. These cases were all associated with the initiation of lithium and responded to treatment with antihistamines, steroids or lithium dosage reduction. Posey [25] described a patient with an intensely pruritic papular dermatitis on her elbows. The pruritus was effectively treated with sulfoxone sodium but the patient's serum lithium level rapidly fell to 0.2 mEq/l from a steady state of 0.8 mEq/l and her mania was exacerbated. Localized pruritic lesions resulting in lichen simplex chronicus have also been reported [26].

A single case of exfoliative dermatitis has been reported in a 16-year-old boy treated with lithium. He initially developed a maculopapular rash 2 weeks after initiation of lithium which progressed to exfoliative dermatitis involving his entire skin surface and his mucous membranes. The condition resolved when lithium was withdrawn but recurred during a second trial of the medication [27]. Such severe reactions appear to be rare but require immediate intervention and are an indication that other psychotropic medications should be used to treat the existing psychiatric disorder.

Two other less-common dermatological conditions associated with lithium are Darier's disease and a lupus-like illness. Darier's disease is a rare, hereditary skin disorder characterized by hyperkeratosis and inflammation. Two cases have been reported of patients with pre-existing Darier's disease which was severely exacerbated after initiation of lithium for coexisting psychiatric conditions. In both cases the Darier's improved with conventional therapies after lithium was discontinued and worsened again during subsequent exposure to lithium. The proposed mechanism is, again, decreased cyclic AMP activity secondary to lithium administration that increases the proliferation rate of epidermal cells [28, 29].

Lithium has also been implicated in a lupus-like syndrome. There is one case report of a lithium-treated patient who developed a malar rash as well as a rash of her abdomen and neck while being treated with lithium. This case is unusual because drug-induced lupus is rarely characterized by physical findings but rather is most often limited to laboratory abnormalities. Laboratory findings in this case included a positive antinuclear antibody titer, mildly elevated sedimentation rate, and a high eosinophil count. Complement, rheumatoid factor, histone antibodies, and other immunological markers were all negative and consistent with a drug-induced lupus. The rash resolved and ANA titer decreased when lithium was discontinued [30].

Other conditions related to lithium treatment include exacerbation of warts with rapid growth and a psoriasiform appearance that eventually required excision [31]. Discoloration of toenails when lithium serum levels are highly therapeutic has also been reported. After lithium levels were reduced slightly, the new nail growth exhibited normal coloration [32].

Antipsychotic Medications

The phenothiazines, especially chlorpromazine, have been implicated in a variety of cutaneous reactions including hypersensitivity, photosensitivity, blue-gray pigmentation and drug-induced lupus-like illness. Five percent of patients receiving chlorpromazine develop cutaneous reactions during treatment [33–43].

The spectrum of hypersensitivity reactions to phenothiazines include urticarial, maculopapular, petechial and edematous reactions. They typically develop between the 1st and 5th weeks of therapy and lesions usually resolve after the medication is discontinued. Provocative tests are sometimes negative and the suspected phenothiazine may be well tolerated after the initial episode of hypersensitivity [33].

Photosensitivity has also been widely reported as a side effect of chronic, high-dose phenothiazine therapy. Again, chlorpromazine is the most commonly implicated member of this class because its cytotoxic metabolite can damage the dermal cell membrane [34]. Photosensitivity reactions have mainly been reported in patients on chlorpromazine doses greater than 600 mg/day [34]. Affected patients have increased pigmentation of sun-exposed skin, most typically on the face, forearms and hands. Studies have shown that unexposed skin also has increased melanin content [35]. The reaction is more commonly observed in women and individuals with light brown hair. The pigmentary changes usually begin in the late spring after the first exposure to sunlight and can look like a tan, however the darkening is progressive and only fades slightly during the winter months. The pigmentary changes generally recur if a phenothiazine is restarted and a patient's skin is not protected against the sun. Even when a phenothiazine is discontinued, hyperpigmentation is occasionally irreversible. In severe cases, patients can go on to develop a blue-gray skin discoloration particularly of the face [36].

General recommendations for managing chlorpromazine photosensitivity include sun avoidance, proper dress, sun block, and phenothiazine dosage reduction. An alternate approach is to change patients from chlorpromazine to other neuroleptics less likely to cause hyperpigmentation. Recently, more research has been done in this area and one report describes 15 patients with chlorpromazine-induced abnormal skin pigmentation who were switched to other neuroleptics. Their symptoms completely resolved over a period of 6 months to 5 years. This study suggests that patients who develop chlorpromazine-induced pigmentary changes should be managed by switching to a non-phenothiazine neuroleptic [37].

Several mechanisms for chlorpromazine photosensitivity have been proposed. Generally, hyperpigmentation is known to be the result of excess melanin synthesis which is determined by an imbalance of darkening and lightening factors. Chlorpromazine appears to affect the balance between darkening factors, including melanocyte-stimulating hormone, androgens and estrogens and lightening factors, specifically epinephrine, norepinephrine and melatonin [36]. Chlorpromazine has also been shown to bind to plasma protein, microsomes and nuclear DNA. Johnson [34] proposed that the mechanism for hyperpigmentation is at the cellular level where a cytotoxic photoproduct acts on the plasma membrane of the dermal and epidermal cell leading to photosensitization. And, finally, a related theory proposes that chlorpromazine forms long-lived free radicals that cause photosensitivity by interacting with cell membranes [38].

There are also multiple explanations for the gray-blue discoloration of the skin which chlorpromazine can cause. One theory proposes pseudomelanin is produced by the interaction of melanin and free radicals in the skin. Other hypotheses assert that affected patients may have defective conjugating pathways for chlorpromazine or that melanin accumulates in phagocytes in the dermis accounting for hyperpigmentation [35].

Chlorpromazine, and more uncommonly the phenothiazines perphenazine and thioridazine, have been infrequently associated with a syndrome resembling systemic lupus erythematosus [39]. Patients with this illnes have a variety of cutaneous symptoms including malar rash, photosensitivity, alopecia and Raynaud's phenomenon [40]. The laboratory profile of this disorder includes positive antinuclear antibody titer, absence of antibody against double-stranded DNA and normal complement levels. As opposed to idiopathic lupus, drug-induced lupus, including that caused by chlorpromazine, is characterized by the following studies: increased serum IgM levels, prolongation of PTT, circulating antibodies against coagulation factors, and a histopathological pattern showing hyperkeratosis, liquefaction degeneration of the basal cells, pigment descending to the upper dermis and patchy lymphocytic infiltration [39]. One theory to explain the occurrence of this lupus-like syndrome proposes that the chlorpromazine acts in a fashion similar to an immunostimulant and signals B and T cells to produce this autoimmune condition [42].

Patients who develop lupus-like illness have usually been treated with chlorpromazine (approximately 400–800 mg/day) for a period of years [39, 41]. Chlorpromazine re-exposures have not been attempted in these patients. Generally, the process is reversible when the chlorpromazine is discontinued. The neuroleptic must be discontinued as soon as the diagnosis is made since patients are at risk of developing serious complications of this lupus-like disorder including bilateral pleural effusions. If necessary, another class of neuroleptic medication should be used to treat the patient.

Antidepressants

Dermatologic side effects from antidepressants are not uncommon. When they do occur, these reactions effects must be promptly recognized and proper management instituted. Allergic reactions that induce urticaria, angioedema, purpura, and exfoliative dermatitis can occur when patients are exposed to tricyclic antidepressants [43]. The tricyclic antidepressant, desipramine seems to induce a higher rate of allergic reactions that other tricyclics with from 2.9–4.2% of patients treated with either desipramine or imipramine developing drug-induced urticaria [44, 45]. Pohl et al. [45] proposed that this phenomenon was due to an allergy to tartrazine, or the Yellow Dye No. 5 contained in tablets of desipramine. Other authors have reported similar dermatological reactions in patients treated with tartrazine-free desipramine [46, 47]. In the most recent study on tartrazine, Bajwa and Asnis [44] administered active desipramine and placebo, both containing tartrazine, to 70 outpatients who met the criteria for major depression. Patients who developed urticaria did so only on the pill containing desipramine. The authors conclude that desipramine alone is responsible for urticaria.

Urticaria usually occurs in the third week of drug administration and at or near therapeutic blood levels. Lowering the dose of desipramine does not appear to be effective in managing urticaria. Instead, one should either attempt treatment with antihistamines such as cyproheptadine or hydroxyzine or discontinue the offending medication altogether. Importantly, there is no cross-allergenicity among various tricyclic antidepressants so another tricyclic can be initiated upon drug discontinuation [48]. Obviously, imipramine, whose major metabolite is desipramine, should be avoided in cases of allergic response to desipramine.

Erythema multiforme is another dermatologic reaction to antidepressant medications; one which needs to be taken quite seriously by the clinician. This disorder comes in two forms. The mild variant is an acute, self-limited syndrome with distinctive, macular-papular eruptions with erythematous scaly plaques, and with or without mucosal erosions [49]. The lesions favor the distal parts of the limbs with involvement of the dorsum of the hands as well as the soles of the feet. The severe variant of erythema multiforme known as the Stevens and Johnson syndrome is more progressive and potentially fatal [50]. Erythema multiforme usually appears after 7–14 days of drug exposure, but can occur within hours for individuals who have been previously exposed to the offending agent. The reaction has been reported to occur with exposure to two different antidepressant medications – trazodone and minaserin [51, 52]. While other antidepressants do not seem to be implicated in the occurrence of this disorder, clinicians should be wary of its possible onset. Management consists of prompt discontinuation of the medication. Rechallenge with the offending agent should not be attempted.

Leukocytoplastic vasculitis is another rarer dermatologic syndrome that should be of concern to the clinician who is administering antidepressant medication. This condition is characterized by inflammation and destruction of small blood vessels [55]. The skin lesions can range from classical palpable purpura to severe ulcerations. Spread to the renal, pulmonary, cardiovascular, hepatic and central nervous systems has been reported. Besides the antidepressant agents trazodone and maprotiline, other agents such aspirin, sulfonamides, iodides, phenothiazines and barbiturates can induce this disorder [53, 54]. This underscores the importance of clinicians always obtaining thorough drug sensitivity histories prior to prescribing any psychotropic agents. As with erythema multiforme, the optimal management for the occurrence of cutaneous vasculitis is drug discontinuation.

Like the phenothiazines, several antidepressant agents have been reported to induce photosensitive skin reactions. Phenelzine, an MAO inhibitor, has been reported to produce a photosensitive reaction. A 39-year-old female developed a confluent macular erythema over her forehead and malar regions, and the sun-exposed area of her upper chest after 1 year of phenelzine [55]. Clomipramine and imipramine have also been reported to produce photosensitive lesions [56, 57]. Several mechanisms have been proposed for these reactions and include: the formation of potentially toxic photosensitive drug products produced in the skin by ultraviolet light; the formation by the drug or its metabolites of complexes with nucleic acids which are then bound in the skin; or a photoallergy directly produced by the parent drug. Photosensitive reactions are managed by discontinuation of the drug and protection from sun exposure.

Two other dermatological conditions less commonly attributable to antidepressants than they are to lithium administration deserve mention. Pustular psoriasis has been reported to be induced by trazodone [58]. The hypothesized mechanism for action is similar to lithium's proposed mechanism for inducing psoriasis, namely inhibition of cyclic AMP activity. And, finally, alopecia has been reported to have occurred with both imipramine and fluoxetine usage [59, 60].

Anticonvulsants

Anticonvulsants, particularly carbamazepine and valproic acid, are being used with increasing frequency in the psychiatric treatment of complicated bipolar disorders [60, 61]. Both of these agents have been noted to have dermatological side effects about which the clinician should be aware. Pruritic rashes have been noted to occur with carbamazepine usage and may usher in other side effects including leukopenia [61]. Rarely, potentially life-threatening exfoliative dermatitis and systemic lupus erythematosus have been reported to have occurred as a result of carbamazepine [63, 64]. Carbamazepine has also been reported to induce hair loss of the telogen effluvium type [65]. This type of alopecia occurs when a disproportionate number of follicles simultaneously enter the telogen or resting stage of the hair cycle immediately preceding loss. Like other dermatologic reactions to carbamazepine, this alopecia is reversible when the medication is discontinued.

Valproic acid has also been reported to induce a variety of dermatologic reactions. Hair loss has been reported to occur in 0.5% of patients reviewed in 41 separate studies [66]. This condition is usually temporary and does not necessarily warrant drug discontinuation. One report suggests that valproic acid may even be responsible for changing hair color in some patients [67]. More serious forms of skin disorders such as scleroderma, cutaneous vasculitis, and lupus erythematosus have been induced by valproic acid [68–70]. As is the case with carbamazepine, should skin reactions to valproic acid occur, the clinician should consider discontinuing the drug and utilizing another medication.

Benzodiazepines

In general, benzodiazepines have few cutaneous side effects, although mild, generalized skin eruptions and photosensitivity have been described [71–74]. Specifically, chlordiazepoxide has been reported to cause dermatological side effects; in one study 2 of 104 patients developed a mild generalized skin eruption. The medication was discontinued shortly afterwards in both cases because of a lack of clinical response [71].

Photosensitivity has also been described in a case report of a patient treated with chlordiazepoxide who developed a moderately severe eczematous reaction involving exposed skin, feet and mucous membranes 2 days after sun exposure. These lesions were treated with cold tap water, diphenhydramine and sun avoidance and cleared within 10 days. When the patient was subsequently rechallenged, the symptoms reappeared [72].

Alprazolam has also been implicated in photosensitivity with the report of a patient who developed itching, redness and scaling of his face a day after a single dose. This condition was treated with topical steroids and sun avoidance. A subsequent alprazolam rechallenge was positive [73].

The precise mechanism of benzodiazepine photosensitivity is unknown. The general theory concerning drug-induced photosensitivity proposes light provides the energy to convert a drug into a compound with allergenic properties which is then capable of causing an allergic reaction without light [74].

Psychotropic Medications and the Treatment of Dermatological Disorders

Psychotropic medications have been used for many years to treat patients with psychiatric disorders who also have chronic skin conditions. More recently, these medications have been recognized as effective therapy for dermatologic diseases such as urticaria and pruritus in patients without coexisting psychiatric problems [75–85].

The antidepressants, in particular doxepin, are the psychotropic medications most commonly used to treat primary cutaneous disease. Most antidepressants have antihistaminic properties and bind to the H1 and H2 receptors which are found on dermal blood vessels. For example, doxepin is an impressive H1 blocker, thought to be 800 times more potent than diphenhydramine [86]. Doxepin also acts as an H2 blocker and is considered to be six times more potent then cimetadine [75]. Trimipramine and amitriptyline are two other antidepressants with significant antihistaminic activity that have been used to treat dermatologic conditions. When antidepressants are compared to conventional antihistamines, they have the distinct advantage of causing less sedation resulting in better patient compliance. The side effects reported on the low dose of doxepin used to treat dermatologic diseases included dry mouth and, less frequently, weight gain [77].

Several studies have addressed the use of doxepin in chronic urticaria, a condition where the symptoms persist for at least 6 weeks. Since an etiology is found in only 30% of the cases, symptoms are typically treated empirically. Greene et al. [77] performed a double-blind, crossover study comparing 10 mg of doxepin three times a day to 25 mg diphenhydramine thrice daily. This series of 50 patients clearly demonstrated the relative efficacy of doxepin over diphenylhydramine. The authors concluded that low-dose doxepin was efficacious in the treatment of chronic urticaria mainly because of its peripheral antihistaminic effect. They also proposed that there may be a central effect of the drug. Since it is generally recognized that emotional disturbances lower the threshold for the development of urticaria, it is possible that patients who respond to doxepin have a subclinical depression or another psychiatric disturbance. Other investigators dispute that doxepin has any central action. They point to the fact that urticaria responds relatively rapidly, weeks before doxepin is known to effect mood, the dose is subtherapeutic and that antidepressants are thought to have little effect on persons without clinical depression [78].

Neittaanmaki et al. [79] described a randomized double-blind trial of doxepin, cinnarizine, cyproheptadine and hydroxyzine in idiopathic cold urticaria and found doxepin to be the most effective medication with the fewest side effects. They subsequently performed an open trial of doxepin in acute and chronic urticaria using higher doses (25–50 mg t.i.d.) and reported that episodes of urticaria were less frequent.

Antidepressants have also been used to treat nocturnal scratching in atopic eczema. Savin et al. [8] performed a double-blind study of trimipramine maleate, trimeprazine tartrate and placebo. They found that neither medication prevented scratching during waking hours but that patients on trimipramine, which has no known antipruritic effect, tended to scratch less often and for shorter periods of time during the first 6 h of sleep. They concluded that this antidepressant improved the overall quality of sleep and therefore led to modest improvements of nocturnal scratching, and dismissed the possibility that trimipramine had treated a subclinical depression because the low dose (50 mg q.h.s.) and rapid improvement in sleep occurred well before an antidepressant effect could be expected.

There are several other skin conditions where psychotropic medications are believed to be efficacious. Recently, lithium has been reported to have an antiviral effect which may possibly be useful in treating herpes simplex infections [81, 82]. Several case reports have described patients whose oral herpes simplex improved when lithium was used to treat their coexisting psychiatric disorder [81]. Amsterdam et al. [82] investigated the antiviral effect of lithium when they performed a retrospective study of 177 patients receiving long-term lithium therapy and found a significant reduction in recurrent herpes infections as compared to controls. However, this study is inconclusive because of its retrospective nature and the generally accepted belief that psychiatric patients have fewer herpes outbreaks when euthymic. Further work needs to be done to explore the usefulness of lithium for herpes simplex in patients without coexisting psychiatric disorders.

A series of three case reports suggests that phenelzine may help aphthous ulcers. Rosenthal [83] reported on 2 of his patients who were given phenelzine for coexisting psychiatric illness whose previously treatment-refractory lesions completely resolved on the monoamine oxidase inhibitor. He then placed the son of one of these patients, who also had severe aphthous ulcers, on phenelzine, and his lesions cleared. When his 2 patients discontinued the phenelzine, their ulcers reappeared.

Preliminary reports indicate that topical chlorpromazine may be an effective treatment for diffuse cutaneous leishmaniasis [84]. Henriksen [84] reported on 3 patients with this intractable parasitic disease who responded to a 2% chlorpromazine ointment. He based his in vivo trial on the in vitro work of Pearson et al. [85] who demonstrated that chlorpromazine killed the protozoan *Leishmania donovania* in hamsters. Pearson et al. [85] proposed that chlorpromazine forms free radicals that act on the protozoal membrane. Further research needs to be done in order to determine if this approach is feasible and if systemic chlorpromazine may be effective in the treatment of this disorder.

Use of Psychotropic Medications in Psychiatric Disorders with Cutaneous Manifestations

Two psychiatric disorders with predominant cutaneous manifestations are included in this category. The first is trichotillomania, the compulsive pulling of hair from any part of the body that eventually leads to traction alopecia. The syndrome was first described by Hallopeau [87] in 1889. It is estimated that up to eight million Americans are affected by this disorder [88]. The disorder begins in childhood and seems to occur mainly in adolescent and young women [89]. A wide variety of behavioral, psychodynamic and biological theories have been postulated to explain the mechanisms central to trichotillomania [90]. Likewise, psychotherapeutic treatments ranging from intensive psychotherapy, hypnosis and behavior modification have been offered to these patients with varying results [91–93]. There have been anecdotal reports that psychopharmacological agents such as chlorpromazine, amitriptyline, imipramine, and isocarboxazide have also been effective [94–97]. Basing their hypothesis that the selective serotonin reuptake inhibiting agent clomipramine would be effective in treating trichotillomania because of similarities between this syndrome and obsessive-compulsive disorders, Swedo et al. [98] performed a recent 10-week double-blind crossover comparison between clomipramine and desipramine in the treatment of severe trichotillomania in 13 women. Treatment with clomipramine resulted in greater improvement in symptoms than desipramine as scored by physicians' ratings. The intensity of the compulsion to pull hair was reduced and patients were more likely to be able to resist the urge to pull out their hair while on clomipramine. It seems that clomipramine offers at least good results in the short-term for those patients who had previously been resistant, if not totally refractory, to treatment.

A second important psychiatric disorder with cutaneous manifestations that is subject to psychotropic management is delusions of parasitosis or infestation. In its pure form, delusions of infestation would now be classified as a delusional disorder in DSM-III-R, however the disorder can occur concurrently with a variety of other psychiatric or physical disorders [99]. The patient suffering from this disorder is plagued by hypochondriacal convictions of being infested by parasites [100]. Most often, the patient brings small boxes containing scales, crusts, hairs and other material picked from skin as proof of such infestation. The resultant skin lesions are symmetrically located excoriations and scars caused by the patient's skin digging.

A variety of pharmacologic agents have been utilized to help these patients with their delusions including antidepressants and neuroleptic agents [101, 102]. While the prognosis of the disorder has been guarded in the past, one neuroleptic agent, pimozide, has been reported, through open and double-blind crossover trials, to be particularly effective in decreasing the delusional intensity in the disorder and its associated itching and picking [103–106]. Pimozide may be effective not only because of its dopamine receptor blocking potential, but also its ability to act as an opiate antagonist [107, 108].

Pimozide, when used to treat delusions of infestation, should be initiated at 1–2 mg/day in divided doses and only after a baseline EKG has been performed [109]. Dosage may be increased every other day but not by more than 10 mg/day. The total dose of pimozide should not exceed 20 mg/day. Pimozide can reduce seizure threshold and should be used with caution in patients who have a history of seizure disorder. Other contraindications for its use include blood dyscrasia, Parkinson's disease, prolonged QT syndrome, coadministration with drugs that prolong the QT interval, and CNS vascular insufficiency. Side effects include EKG changes, extrapyramidal syndromes, and in a few instances sudden unexpected deaths. In many patients with delusions of parasitosis, pimozide can be discontinued after 3–5 months of treatment [110].

As outlined in this review, the interaction of the various classes of pyschotropic medications and the skin can have many different presentations, some desirable and others definitely not. Lithium has probably been the most studied in this regard but this medication is clearly not the only psychotropic that affects the skin. Several areas require further study including the use of psychotropic medications for dermatological disorders and more research on other psychiatric disorders with dermatological manifestations.

References

1   Abel EA; DiCicco LM, Orenberg EK, Fraki JE, Farber EM: Drugs in exacerbation of psoriasis. J Am Arch Dermatol 1986;15:1007–1021.
2   Pande AC, Max P, Donnelly RF: Lithium associated with psoriasis. J Clin Psychiatry 1986;47:330.
3   Lowe NJ, Ridgway HB: Generalized pustular psoriasis precipitated by lithium carbonate. Arch Dermatol 1978;114:1788–1789.
4   Skoven I, Thormann J: Lithium compound treatment and psoriasis. Arch Dermatol 1979; 115:1185–1187.
5   Sarantidis D, Waters B: A review and controlled study of cutaneous conditions associated with lithium carbonate. Br J Psychiatry 1983;143:42–50.
6   Evans DL, Martin W: Lithium carbonate and psoriasis. Am J Psychiatry 1979;136:1326–1327.
7   Paragus MG: Lithium adverse reactions in psychiatric patients. Pharmacol Biochem Behav 1984;21:65–69.
8   Lazarus GS, Gilgor RS: Psoriasis, polymorphonuclear leukocytes and lithium carbonate. Arch Dermatol 1979;115:1183–1184.
9   Heng MCY: Cutaneous manifestations of lithium toxicity. Br J Dermatol 1982;106:107–109.
10   Abel EA: Diagnosis of drug-induced psoriasis. Semin Dermatol 1992;11:269–274.
11   Ruiz-Maldonado R, Perez de Francisco C, Tamayo L: Lithium dermatitis. JAMA 1973;224: 1534.
12   Remmer HI, Falk WE: Successful treatment of lithium-induced acne. J Clin Psychiatry 1986;47:48.
13   McGennis AJ: Lithium carbonate and tetracycline interaction. Br Med J 1978;i:1183.
14   Aldoroty NA, LeVine WR: Dermatosis and lithium therapy. Am J Psychiatry 1980;137:870.
15   Kuhnley EJ, Granoff AL: Exfoliative dermatitis during lithium therapy. Am J Psychiatry 1979; 136:1340–1341.
16   Dawber R, Mortimer P: Hair Loss during lithium treatment. Br J Dermatol 1982;107:124–125.
17   Silvestri A, Santonastaso P, Paggiarin D: Alopecia areata during lithium therapy: A case report. Gen Hosp Psych 1988;10:603–604.
18   Orwin A: Hair loss following lithium therapy. Br J Dermatol 1982;108:503–504.
19   McCreadie RG, Morrison DP: The impact of lithium in south-west Scotland. I. Demographic and clinical findings. Br J Psychiatry 1985;146:70–80.
20   Yassa R: Hair loss during lithium therapy. Am J Psychiatry 1986;143:943.
21   Warnock JK: Psychotropic medication and drug-related alopecia. Psychosomatics 1991; 32:149–152.
22   Minuz CE, Salem RB, Director KL: Hair loss in a patient receiving lithium. Psychosomatics 1982;23:312–313.
23   Yassa R, Ananth J: Hair loss in the course of lithium treatment: A report of two cases. Can J Psychiatry 1983;28:132–133.

24 Callaway CL, Hendrie HC, Luby ED: Cutaneous conditions observed in patients during treatment with lithium. Am J Psychiatry 1968;124:1124–1125.
25 Posey RE: Lithum carbonate dermatitis. JAMA 1972;221:1517.
26 Shukla S, Mukherjee S: Lichen simplex chronicus during lithium treatment. Am J Psychiatry 1984;141:909–910.
27 Rifkin A, Kurtin SB, Quitkin F, Klein F: Lithium-induced folliculitis. Am J Psychiatry 1973;130:1018–1019.
28 Clark RD, Hammer CJ, Patterson SD: A cutaneous disorder (Darier's disease) evidently exacerbated by lithium carbonate. Psychosomatics 1986;27:800–801.
29 Milton G, Peck GL, Fu JL, DiGiovanna JJ, Nordlund JJ, Thomas JH, Sanders SF: Exacerbation of Darier's disease by lithium carbonate. J Am Arch Dermatol 1990;23:926–928.
30 Shukla VR, Borison RL: Lithium and lupuslike illness. JAMA 1982;248:921–922.
31 White SW: Lithium and warts. Int J Dermatol 1982;21:107.
32 Hooper JF: Lithium carbonate and toenails. Am J Psychiatry 1981;138:1519.
33 Baldessarini RJ: Drugs and the treatment of psychiatric disorders; in Gilman AJ, Goodman LS, Gilman A (eds): The Pharmacological Basis of Therapeutics. New York, Pergamon Press, 1990, p 401.
34 Johnson BE: Cellular mechanisms of chlorpromazine photosensitivity. Proc R Soc Med 1974;67:871–873.
35 Robins AH: Melanosis after prolonged chlorpromazine therapy. S Afr Med J 1975;49:1521–1524.
36 Bond WS, Yee GC: Ocular and cutaneous effects of chronic phenothiazine therapy. Am J Hosp Pharm 1980;37:74–78.
37 Lal S, Bloom D, Silver B, Desjardins B: Replacement of chlorpromazine with other neuroleptics: effect on abnormal skin pigmentation and ocular changes. J Psychiatry Neurosci 1993;18:173–177.
38 Ljunggren B: Phenothiazine phototoxicity: Toxic chlorpramazine photoproducts. J Invest Dermatol 1977;69:383–386.
39 Pavlidakey GP, Hashimoto K, Heller GL, Daneshvar S: Chlorpromazine-induced lupus-like disease. Am Acad Dermatol 1985;13:109–115.
40 Cush JJ, Goldings EA: Southwestern internal medicine conference: Drug-induced lupus: Clinical spectrum and pathogenesis. Am J Med Sci 1985;290:36–45.
41 Goldman LS, Hudson JI, Weddington WW: Lupus-like illness associated with chlorpromazine. Am J Psychiatry 1980;137:1613–1614.
42 Schoen RT, Trentham DE: Drug-Induced lupus: An adjuvant disease? Am J Med 1981;71:5–8.
43 Warnock JK, Knesevich JW: Adverse cutaneous reactions to antidepressants. Am J Psychiatry 1988;145:425–430.
44 Bajwa WK, Asnis GM: Desipramine-induced urticaria: a clinical problem. J Nerv Ment Dis 1991;179:108–109.
45 Pohl R, Balon R, Berchov R, Yeragani VK: Allergy to tartrazine in antidepressant. Am J Psychiatry 1987;144:237–238.
46 Biederman J, Gonzalez E: Desipramine and cutaneous reactions in pediatric outpatients. J Clin Psychiatry 1988;49:178–182.
47 Hollander E: Non-tartrazine allergy with desipramine. Am J Psychiatry 1987;144:9.
48 Salem R: Lack of cross allergenicity between tricyclic antidepressants. South Med J 1982;8:1020–1021.
49 Huff JC, Weston WL, Tonneson MG: Erythema multiforme: A critical review of characteristics, diagnostic criteria, and causes. J Am Acad Dermatol 1983;8:763–775.
50 Stevens AM, Johnson FC: A new eruptive fever associated with stomatitis and ophthalmia. Am J Dis Child 1922;24:526–533.
51 Ford HE, Jenike MA: Erythema multiforme associated with trazodone therapy: Case report. J Clin Psychiatry 1985;6:294–295.
52 Quraishy E: Erythema multiforme during treatment with mianserin: a case report. Br J Dermatol 1981;104:481.

53 Mann SC, Walker MM, Messenger GG, Greenstein RA: Leukocytoclastic vasculits secondary to trazodone treatment. J Am Acad Dermatol 1984;10:669–670.

54 Oakley AMM, Hodge L: Cutaneous vasculitis from maprotiline. Aust NZ J Med 1985;15:256–257.

55 Case JD, Yusk JW, Callen JP: Photosensitive reaction to phenelzine: A case report. Photodermatology 1988;5:101–102.

56 Tunca Z, Tunca MI, Dilsiz A, Bayou U, Hancioglu M: Clomipramine induced pseudocyanotic pigmentation. Am J Psychiatry 1989;146:552–553.

57 Walter-Ryan WG, Kern EE, Shiriff JR, Thomas JM: Persistent Photoaggravated cutaneous eruption induced by imipramine. JAMA 1985;254:357–358.

58 Barth JH, Baker H: Generalized pustular psoriasis precipitated by trazodone in the treatment of depression. Br J Dermatol 1986;115:629–630.

59 Baral J, Deakins S: Imipramine induced alopecia areata like lesions. J Am Acad Dermatol 1987;26:198.

60 Jenike MA: Fluoxetine induced hair loss. Am J Psychiatry 1991;148:392.

61 Ballenger JC, Post RM: Carbamazepine in manic depressive illness: A new treatment. Am J Psychiatry 1980;137:782–790.

62 Pope HG: Valproic acid for the treatment of mania. Curr Affective Dis 1991;10:5–13.

63 Ford B, Bieder L: Exfoliative dermatitis due to carbamazepine. N Z Med J 1968;68:386–387.

64 Oner A, Topaloglu R, Besbas N, Topaloglu H: Carbamazepine induced systemic lupus erythematosus: another warning. Clin Neurol Neurosurg 1990;92:261–262.

65 Shuper A, Stahl B, Weitz R: Carbamazepine induced hair loss. Drug Intell Clin Pharm 1985;19:924.

66 Lewis JR: Valproic acid: A new anticonvulsant agent. JAMA 1978;240:2190–2192.

67 Herranz JL, Artega R, Armijo JA: Change in hair color induced by valproic acid. Dev Med Child Neurol 1981;23:386–387.

68 Bleck TP, Smith MC: Possible induction of systemic lupus erythematosus by valproate. Epilepsia 1990;31:343–345.

69 Kamper AM, Valentijn RM, Strickler BH, Purcell PM: Cutaneous vasculitis induced by sodium valproate. Lancet 1991;337:497–498.

70 Goihman-Yahr M, Leal G, Essenfeld-Yahr E: Generalized morphea: A side effect of valproate sodium? Arch Dermatol 1980;116:621.

71 Tobin JM, Lewis NDC: New psychotherapeutic agent, chlordiazepine. JAMA 1959;174:1242–1249.

72 Luton EF, Finchum RN: Photosensitivity reaction to chlordiazepoxide. Arch Dermatol 1965;91:362–363.

73 Kanwar AJ, Gupta R, Das Mehta S: Photosensitivity due to alprazolam. Dermatologica 1990;181:75.

74 Baer RL, Harber LC: Photosensitivity to drugs. Arch Dermatol 1961;83:7–10.

75 Gupta MA, Gupta AK, Ellis CN: Antidepressants drugs in dermatology. Arch Dermatol 1987;123:647–652.

76 Newbold PCH: Antidepressants and skin disease. Br Med J 1988;296–379.

77 Greene SL, Reed CE, Schroeter AL: Double-blind crossover study comparing doxepin with diphenhydramine for the treatment of chronic urticaria. J Am Acad Dermatol 1985;12:669–675.

78 Ledo A, Harto A, Sendagorta E: Doxepin in the treatment of chronic urticaria. J Am Acad Dermatol 1985;13:1058–1059.

79 Neittaanmaki H, Myohanen T, Fraki JE: Comparison of cinnarizine, cyproheptadine, doxepin and hydroxyzine in treatment of idiopathic cold urticaria: Usefulness of doxepin. J Am Acad Dermatol 1984;11:483–489.

80 Savin JA, Paterson WD, Adam K, Oswald I: Effects of trimeprazine and trimipramine on nocturnal scratching with atopic eczema. Arch Dermatol 1979;115:313–315.

81 Gillis A: Lithium in herpes simplex. Lancet 1983;ii:516.

82 Amsterdam JD, Maislin G, Rybakowski J: A possible antiviral action of lithium carbonate in herpes simplex virus infections. Biol Psychiatry 1990;27:447–453.

83 Rosenthal SH: Does phenelzine relieve aphthous ulcers of the mouth? N Engl J Med 1984; 311:1442.

84 Henriksen T: Treatment of diffuse cutaneous leishmaniasis with chlorpromazine ointment. Lancet 1983;i:126.

85 Pearson RD, Manian AA, Harcus JL, Hall D, Hewlett EL: Lethal effect of phenothiazine neuroleptics on the pathogenic protozoan *Leishmania donovani*. Science 1982;217:369–371.

86 Richelson E: Tricyclic antidepressants and neurotransmitter receptors. Psychiatr Ann 1979;9: 186–195.

87 Hallopeau M: Alopécie par grattage (trichomanie ou trichotillomanie). Ann Dérmatol Vénérol 1889;10:440–401.

88 Arzin NH, Nunn RG: Habit Control in a Day. New York, Simon & Schuster, 1978.

89 Muller SA: Trichotillomania. Dermatol Clin 1987;5:595–601.

90 Stein DJ, Hollander E: Dermatology and conditions related to obsessive-compulsive disorder. J Am Acad Dermatol 1992;26:237–42.

91 Krishnan KRR, Davidson JR, Guajardo C: Trichotillomania: A review. Compr Psychiatry 1985; 26:123–128.

92 Gardnes GG: Hypnotherapy in the management of childhood habit disorders. J Pediatr 1978; 92:838–840.

93 de L'Horne DJ: Behavior therapy for trichotillomania. Behav Res Ther 1977;15:192–196.

94 Childers RT: Report of two cases of trichotillomania of long standing duration and their response to chlorpromazine. J Clin Exp Psychopathol 1958;19:141–144.

95 Snyder S: Trichotillomania treated with amitriptyline. J Nerv Ment Dis 1980;168:505–507.

96 Sachdeva JS, Sidhu BS: Trichotillomania associated with depression. J Indian Med Assoc 1987;85:151–152.

97 Krishnan RR, Davidson J, Miller R: MAO inhibitor therapy in trichotillomania associated with depression: A case report. J Clin Psychiatry 1984;45:267–268.

98 Swedo S et al: A double-blind comparison of clomipramine and desipramine in the treatment of trichotillomania (hair pulling). N Engl J Med 1989;321:497–501.

99 Diagnostic and Statistical Manual of Mental Disorders: DSM-III-R, ed 3, rev. Washington, American Psychiatric Association, 1987.

100 Lynch PJ: Delusions of parasitosis. Semin Dermatol 1993;12:39–45.

101 Frithz A: Delusions of infestation: Treatment by depot injections of neuroleptics. Clin Exp Dermatol 1979;4:194.

102 Munro A: Monosymptomatic hypochondriacal psychosis manifesting as delusions of parasitosis. Arch Dermatol 1978;114:940.

103 Reilly TM: Pimozide in monosymptomatic psychosis. Lancet 1975;i:1385.

104 Reilly TM, Jopling WH, Beard AW: Successful treatment with pimozide of delusional parasitosis. Br J Dermatol 1978;98:457.

105 Riding J, Munro A: Pimozide in the treatment of monosymptomatic hypochondrial psychosis. Acta Psychiatr Scand 1975;52:23.

106 Hamann K, Avnstorp C: Delusions of infestation treated by pimozide: A double-blind crossover clinical study. Acta Dermatovener 1982;62:55–58.

107 Johnson GC, Anton RF: Pimozide in delusions of parasitosis. J Dermatovener 1982;62:55–58.

108 Johnson GC, Anton RF: Pimozide in delusions of parasitosis. J Clin Psychiatry 1983;44:233.

109 Damiani JT, Flowers FP, Pierce DK: Pimozide in delusions of parasitosis. J Am Acad Dermatol 1990;22:312–313.

110 Lindskov R, Badsgaard O: Delusions of infestation treated with pimozide: A follow-up study. Acta Derm Venereol 1985;65:267–270.

Dr. Richard L. Goldberg, Department of Psychiatry, Georgetown University Medical Center, 3800 Reservoir Road, NW, Washington, DC 20007-2197 (USA)

Silver PA (ed): Psychotropic Drug Use in the Medically Ill.
Adv Psychosom Med. Basel, Karger, 1994, vol 21, pp 107–137

Psychotropic Medications in Oncology and in AIDS Patients

Steven Bluestine, Lynna Lesko

Memorial Sloan-Kettering Cancer Center, New York, N. Y., USA

Introduction

Prevalence of Cancer

In 1986, approximately 930,000 people were diagnosed with cancer. Of the 43 million Americans now living, 30% will develop some form of malignancy and 3 of 4 families will be affected. However, data from the National Cancer Institute shows that cancer deaths have been declining since 1966 [1]. This change is due to more rigorous treatments, frequently involving multiple modalities (chemotherapy, surgery, and radiation), multidrug regimens, and innovative procedures such as bone marrow transplantation. As a result of these advances, 4 of 10 patients who got cancer in 1987 will be surviving the illness 5 years after the diagnosis. However, with longer patient survival, there are more delayed effects of treatment.

With the shift of perception from an invariably rapidly progressive, debilitating, and fatal disease to an illness with a more chronic course and a potential for cure or long-term remission, there has been a shift in psychiatric attitudes as well. Attention was formerly focused largely on death and dying issues; now there is also attention paid to quality of life issues and effects of treatment regimens (both immediate and delayed). Patients no longer accepts global statement such as 'you should be grateful just to be alive'. In this setting, psychotropic medications have received special attention, since they have the potential to effect rapid change in patient's mental state, comfort, well-being, and quality of life. With their increased use, there has also come increased awareness of the need to use them differently in the cancer population as compared with the medically healthy.

This chapter will review the normal range of responses to cancer, the most frequently encountered psychiatric disorders and their pharmacologic treatment, and several special topics such as side effects of specific cancer treatments, nausea and vomiting, anorexia, pain, and *advanced* AIDS. The *early* neurologic manifestations of AIDS are discussed by Trinidad and Silver [this vol.].

Prevalence of Disorders

There are many myths about the prevalence of psychiatric distress and psychiatric illness among patients with cancer. These have ranged from 'patients manage well and only a few need help' to 'all patients are depressed and need intensive psychiatric intervention'. Prevalence studies have not supported either of these extremes. The Psychosocial Collaborative Oncology Group (PSYCOG) reported a study of 215 randomly selected hospitalized and ambulatory patients at three major cancer centers [2]. Their findings are summarized in figure 1. Using DSM-III criteria, they found that 47% of patients met the criteria for a psychiatric disorder and 53% did not. Of the 47% with recognizable psychiatric disorder, 68% had an adjustment disorder with depressed, anxious, or mixed mood; the spectrum of depressive disorders, including adjustment disorder with depressed mood and major depression, accounted for the majority of diagnoses (81%).

Nearly 90% of the psychiatric disorders observed were either reactions to or manifestation of the treatment. Only 11% represented prior psychiatric problems, such as anxiety disorders, panic attacks, or personality disorders. Patients with cancer are thus largely psychologically healthy individuals who usually have emotional distress syndromes related to illness.

Principles of Psychiatric Medication Usage in Cancer Patients

Several basic principles should be kept in mind when using psychiatric mediations in patients with cancer. While there have been few clinical research studies of psychotropic medications in cancer patients, clinical experience suggests these five important rules:

(1) Start with a lower dose than would ordinarily be used in a physically healthy patient. (2) Increase the dosage of the drug more slowly than would be customary with a physically healthy patient. (3) The therapeutic dose needed for a medically ill patient may be significantly lower than for a physically

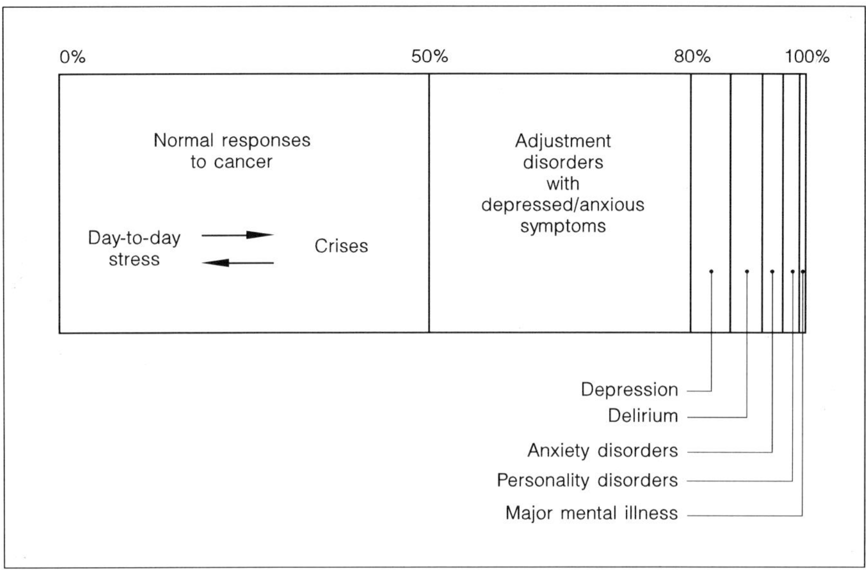

Fig. 1. Spectrum of psychiatric disorders in cancer. 'Major mental illness' refers to schizophrenia and bipolar disorder. Derived from Derogatis et al. [2].

healthy patient. (4) Be aware of the major side effects of the drug being used, and how they may have a deleterious effect on an organ system related to tumor site or treatment. Examples of this include anticholinergic effects of tricyclic antidepressants in a patient with urinary retention or one on high doses of narcotics; the potentially lethal interaction of serotonin reuptake inhibitors with monoamine oxidase inhibitors, including the antineoplastic agent procarbazine; or the potential renal toxicity in a patient being treated with cisplatin and lithium. (5) Treat to ameliorate symptoms and improve comfort, rather than on the basis of diagnosis. For example, assuming there is no contraindication, a sedating tricyclic antidepressant may help a patient with insomnia and anorexia even if they do not meet the full criteria for a major depressive episode.

Treatment of Various Psychiatric Disorders

Anxiety

Anxiety in the cancer setting is usually of two basic types: acute, related to cancer and its treatment, and chronic, related to anxiety disorders that predate the cancer diagnosis but are exacerbated during the illness. Acute anxiety in response to stress can occur at many points during cancer treatment. These points are listed as follows: (1) While awaiting the cancer diagnosis. (2) While awaiting procedures associated with pain such as lumbar puncture, wound debridement, or bone marrow aspiration and biopsy. (3) Prior to major treatments such as chemotherapy or radiation. (4) While awaiting test results. (5) When treatment plans or regimens are changed. (6) In anticipation of termination of treatment. (7) On the anniversary of cancer events. (8) After learning of relapse or change in prognosis. These anxiety states are best managed with a combination of supportive therapy, pharmacotherapy, and behavioral therapy.

Other causes of acute anxiety are poorly controlled pain, hypoxia, endocrine abnormalities, medications such as steroids or theophylline, and drug withdrawal from CNS depressants such as alcohol, barbiturates, benzodiazepines, and narcotics. Akathisia due to neuroleptics is frequently mistaken for anxiety. Mention should also be made of the fact that a pulmonary embolus can present with sudden onset of 'anxiety' with a primary complaint of dyspnea, and should be considered in the differential diagnosis of a newly anxious patient. While anxiolytics are often used as adjuncts in managing these conditions, primary treatment is frequently directed at the underlying cause.

Chronic anxiety states that may be exacerbated or cause problems during cancer include phobias (particularly needle phobias and claustrophobia in diagnostic imaging equipment), generalized anxiety disorder, and panic disorders. These conditions may require the use of anxiolytic medications, supplemented in many cases with behavioral techniques (relaxation, systematic desensitization, or hypnosis).

The usual pharmacologic treatment for anxiety, both acute and chronic, is with benzodiazepines. These medications are safe and effective in the cancer population. A variety of agents is available, and selection is based on several factors, such as route of administration, presence or absence of active metabolites, and half-life. Lorazepam is the only agent available in both a reliably absorbed parenteral form and an oral form; this makes it very useful for patients who will be unable to take oral medications for part or all of their treatment because of stomatitis, esophagitis, surgery, etc. Lorazepam, oxazepam, and temazepam are metabolized by conjugation, which makes them safer to use in patients with liver impairment than other benzodiazepines, which are metabolized by oxidation. Short-acting agents, such as lorazepam, oxazepam, and alprazolam must be given three to four times per day, while long-acting agents such as chlordiazepoxide, diazepam, clorazepate, and clonazepam have active metabolites and thus can usually be given twice per day in chronic administration. However, their long half-life increases the risk of accumulation, especially in the elderly and patients with altered hepatic function.

Initial doses of benzodiazepines vary with the potency of the agent used. Common starting doses are 0.25–0.5 mg t.i.d. of alprazolam, 0.5–1.0 mg t.i.d. of lorazepam. 5–10 mg b.i.d. of diazepam, or 0.5–1.0 mg b.i.d. of clonazepam. The dosage can then be increased every 1–2 days until relief is obtained. If a patient experiences anxiety between doses (common with shorter-acting agents such as alprazolam), the frequency may need to be increased or a longer-acting agent substituted. Patients with situational anxiety may only need to take medication at specific times, such as prior to a procedure or on the day they come to the clinic. On the other hand, patients with more long-standing anxiety should be given anxiolytics on a 24-hour schedule, since an 'on request' order places an additional burden on the already anxious patient. It is important to give an adequate dose of benzodiazepine to relieve anxiety; while patients who have been on benzodiazepines for long periods need to be tapered rather than abruptly stopped [3], fears of addiction in the cancer population are exaggerated [4].

The use of barbiturates and meprobamate for anxiety in cancer has largely been supplanted by the benzodiazepines, with their greater efficacy and higher margin of safety. Of particular concern in medically ill patients is the greater incidence of hypotension and respiratory depression with barbiturates and meprobamate.

Antipsychotics are not indicated for first-line treatment of anxiety, but they can be very useful if benzodiazepines are not efficacious. They are the first choice in our center for treating anxiety that is felt to be due to organic mental syndrome such as delirium, since benzodiazepines frequently worsen confusion in the medically ill [5]. Some prefer benzodiazepines in this situation because they are physiologically more benign; however, the doses of neuroleptics used for anxiety (such as 10–50 mg thioridazine or 0.5–3 mg haloperidol per day) are much lower than for treating psychosis in physically healthy individuals. Sedating neuroleptics, such as thioridazine or chlorpromazine, are usually preferred for use as antianxiety agents, provided that their greater anticholinergic, anti-α-adrenergic, and antihistaminic effects can be tolerated.

Antihistamines such as hydroxyzine or diphenhydramine are occassionally used for their mild antianxiety effects. They are useful in patients where there is a concern about the possible abuse of benzodiazepines, but are largely ineffective as first-line drugs for treating major anxiety situations.

In the ambulatory setting, buspirone is useful for chronic anxiety; it has the advantage of not inducing tolerance or physiologic dependence. Its primary disadvantage is that it must be titrated to an effective dose over a period of several weeks, which makes it somewhat impractical for use in many acute situations in the oncology setting where patients need immediate relief of their symptoms. However, with a cooperative patient it is possible to begin both

Table 1. Thirteen studies of depression in cancer patients

Reference	n	Site and stage	Method	Percentage of depression
Koenig et al. [11]	36	advanced bowel cancer, hospitalized	MMPI	25
Peck and Boland [12]	50	ambulatory radiotherapy patients, all sites and stages	interview	10 severe 32 moderate 32 mild
Hinton [10]	50	terminally ill, referred for psychiatric consultation	interview	58
Craig and Abeloff [13]	30	advanced stage, all sites, hospitalized	SCL-90	50
Plumb and Holland [14]	97	advanced stage, all sites, hospitalized	BDI	4 severe 19 moderate
Levine et al. [15]	100	all stages and sites, hospitalized, referred for psychiatric consultation	interview; DSM-III criteria	56
Massie et al. [16]	334	all stages and sites, ambulatory and hospitalized, referred for psychiatric consultation	interview; DSM-III criteria	49 (includes adjustment disorder with depressed mood)
Plumb and Holland [17]	80	all sites, advanced stage, hospitalized	structured interview, current and past, Psychologic Adjustment Scale	20
Derogatis et al. [2]	215	all stages and sites, half ambulatory, half hospitalized	DSM III criteria	13
Bukberg et al. [18]	67	hospitalized in Medical Oncology units	modified DSM-III criteria, eliminating physical symptoms	24 severe 18 moderate 14 some depressive symptoms
Lansky et al. [9]	500	largely ambulatory, all women, breast, bowel, melanoma, gynecological cancer	DSM-III HDS (rated only for non-medically related symptoms) Zung Depression Scale	4.5 (DSM-III) 5.3 (HDS and Zung)
Evans et al. [19]	83	all hospitalized women with gynecological cancer (except ovarian)	DSM-III HDS	23 major depression 24 adjustment disorder with depressed mood
Massie and Holland [20]	564	all sites, all stages, ambulatory and hospitalized	interview; DSM-III criteria	20 major depression 27 adjustment disorder with depressed mood 1 bipolar

MMPI = Minnesota Multiphasic Personality Inventory; SCL-90 = Hopkins Symptom Checklist-90; BDI = Beck Depression Inventory; HDS = Hamilton Depression Scale.
Modified from Massie [21].

buspirone and a benzodiazepine, then taper the benzodiazepine after a therapeutic dosage of buspirone has been achieved.

All benzodiazepines have the potential to depress respiration via a central nervous system mechanism. This effect is most pronounced with intravenous use. It is rarely a problem in clinical practice, except in patients with preexisting respiratory compromise. In cases in which a patient's hyperventilation or sensation of dyspnea and shortness of breath is secondary to anxiety or panic, use of a benzodiazepine will usually ease respiration rather than depress it. In patients with chronic obstructive pulmonary disease or other respiratory difficulty, hydroxyzine may be used, as it has less respiratory depressant effect than benzodiazepines [6].

Behavioral treatment for anxiety is very useful for patients with certain problems, such as needle phobias or panic disorders, and for patients who will not or cannot take medication. Psychotherapy for patients with acute anxiety states focuses on educating patients about procedures, etc., on correcting misperceptions, and on reassurance. Staff education can also be important, especially if a patient's anxiety is great enough to require modification in hospital routines (such as giving a patient anxiolytic medication before every procedure). A detailed discussion of these methods of treatment is beyond the scope of this chapter; good references are the chapters by Massie et al. [7] and Mastrovito [8].

Depression

Depression in cancer patients can result from several causes: stress related to the cancer diagnosis and treatment, medications such as steroids, interferon, or other chemotherapeutic agents, or as an episode of a unipolar or bipolar mood disorder. The prevalence of major depression in cancer patients has varied in different studies, from 4.5% [9] to 58% [10]; the results of these studies are summarized in table 1.

The three most common diagnoses which are made in depressed patients in the cancer setting are adjustment disorder with depressed mood, major depression, and organic mood disorder, depressed. Differentiating among these is important, since it has implications for both illness course and treatment. Since somatic indicators of depression such as changes in sleep, appetite, energy, libido, and psychomotor activity are often affected by cancer or its treatment, these are frequently unreliable in making a diagnosis. Instead, a careful cognitive exam (to rule out delirium), a review of the patient's history and current chart (to look for possible organic causes), and careful questioning about signs and symptoms of major depression that are not usually affected by medical state alone, such as hopelessness, helplessness, guilt, worthlessness, and suicidal ideation, is more helpful. Other factors which will affect treatment deci-

Table 2. Seven trials of antidepressants in cancer patients

References	n	Group studied	Intervention	Outcome
Purohit et al. [22]	39	patients undergoing radiation	imipramine, up to 75 mg p.o. daily	80% of imipramine group improved, as opposed to 42% of the 'nontreated' group
Costa et al. [23]	75	women hospitalized for gynecological cancer	mianserin	the treatment group showed significant improvement on HDS
Maguire et al. [24]	10	women, postmastectomy	cognitive therapy, with and without pharmacotherapy	both groups improved, but there was less relapse in the combined therapy group
Lansky [25]	25	terminally ill patients	nortriptyline	study not completed because of high attention rate (due to antidepressant side effects or progression of disease)
Holland et al. [26]	147	cancer patients both ambulatory ambulatory and hospitalized	alprazalam vs. progressive relation	both groups showed an almost 50% decrease in anxiety and depression, but in the alprazolam group, the effects appeared earlier
Evans et al. [27]	22	women with gynecological cancer	imipramine in two dose schedules	patients treated with adequate doses improved whether the diagnosis was major depressive episode or adjustment disorder with depressed mood
Carrol [28]	20	terminally ill patients	alprazolam	the drug-treated group had significant improvement in HDS

HDS = Hamilton Depression Scale.
Adapted from Mermelstein et al. [29].

sions are the presence of psychotic features (rare unless the depression is caused by steroids), the presence of organic impairment (which suggests a delirium either coexisting with or causing the depression), the patient's level of sedation or agitation, and a history of manic episodes.

The mainstay of treatment for depression in the cancer patient is pharmacotherapy along with supportive follow-up. There are relatively few controlled studies of use of antidepressants in cancer patients (table 2). However, clinical experience indicates that these medications are effective in and well tolerated by patients with cancer. All antidepressants are efficacious for treating depression in the cancer population; selection is based on their side effect profile. Secondary amines such as desipramine and nortriptyline are less sedating and have a lower incidence of anticholinergic side effects. They are therefore indicated if a patient is already on other anticholinergic medications such as pain medications or antiemetics, or if a patient has stomatitis and/or esophagitis which would be exacerbated by the drying effects of anticholinergic agents. If a patient has pain in addition to depression, tertiary amines such as amitriptyline or imipramine may be used since they have been the most studied as analgesic adjuncts [30]. For patients with insomnia, doxepin or amitriptyline may be used as they are the most sedating agents. Although blood levels of several agents can be measured, at this time only nortriptyline has a therapeutic window; this can make it easier to titrate in certain patients who are noncompliant or sensitive to drug side effects.

Tricyclic antidepressants need to be started slowly (such as 10–25 mg nortriptyline or 25 mg desipramine at bedtime) and increased by 10–25 mg/day every 2–3 days. Cancer patients often reach plateaus, at which they have side effects before reaching a full therapeutic dose; they may have to be maintained at this dose for several weeks before they develop enough tolerance to the side effects to increase their dose. In medically ill populations, it has been noted that patients frequently respond to lower than expected doses, such as 25–75 mg nortriptyline or 50–125 mg desipramine per day. With the availability of blood level monitoring of antidepressants, it has also been found that many cancer patients achieve therapeutic levels on these low doses, in addition to tolerating them better than the higher doses commonly used in healthy patients.

As with all patients being considered for tricyclic therapy, there are some preliminary considerations. They should have an EKG to rule out heart block (greater than first degree) or prolongation of the PR interval. Since the most common troublesome side effects are anticholinergic (even with secondary amines), special care should be taken with patients with urinary retention, constipation, stomatitis or esophagitis (caused by chemotherapy or radiation), or other problems which will be exacerbated by this. Orthostatic hypotension is a potentially dangerous side effect, which is not dose related but is more likely to occur in debilitated patients; nortriptyline is the least likely to cause this side effect. Tricyclics vary in sedative activity; with more sedating agents such as amitriptyline and imipramine care must be taken with cancer patients who are taking other sedating agents, such as benzodiazepines, narcotics, anticonvulsants, antiemetics, antihistamines, or neuroleptics.

For patients who have previously shown a good response to monoamine oxidase inhibitors, these can be continued in the cancer setting provided the patient can tolerate their side effects such as orthostatic hypotension, sexual dysfunction, and insomnia. However, they are rarely used as first-line treatment in these patients for several reasons. The dietary restrictions are difficult for patients who are usually having problems with decreased nutritional intake due to their cancer. Many oncologists feel it may be unwarranted to add dietary restrictions for such patients. A more serious problem is the potential for drug interactions. Since cancer patients invariably develop pain, and since they often require emergency care, there is always the possibility that they will inadvertently be given medications which can cause hypertensive crisis (such as sympathomimetic amines) or excitation and hyperpyrexia (such as meperidine or dextromethorphan).

Lithium carbonate is most often used in the depressed cancer patient who has a history of manic episodes. It should be maintained in patients who have been receiving it prior to their cancer diagnosis. Careful monitoring of lithium blood levels, thyroid function (with TSH measurements as well as T4 and T3), and cardiac rhythm with EKG is necessary, especially in periods of altered fluid status such as postoperatively and during aggressive hydration for chemotherapy, and when patients are receiving other nephrotoxic agents such as cisplatin or aminogylcosides. There are several reports in the literature regarding the potential usefulness of lithium for prevention of steroid-induced mood changes [31]. We have found lithium helpful in preventing steroid-related symptoms in a few patients, but prefer to use neuroleptics should symptoms appear. Lithium has been shown to cause neutrophilic leukocytosis due to mobilization of a proportion of polymorphonuclear leukocytes from bone marrow reserves [32]. There was initial enthusiasm that this would be of possible benefit in neutropenic cancer patients, but the functional capabilities of these leukocytes have not been determined.

The newer selective serotonin reuptake inhibitors (SSRIs) are antidepressant agents that have not yet been fully studied in the medically ill. Our clinical experience indicates that they can be used safely and effectively in the ambulatory cancer setting. They have the advantage of being stimulating agents, unlike the tricyclics which are sedating. They are usually well tolerated, particularly in younger patients. However, several of their properties make them difficult to use with other populations. They can cause overstimulation and jitteriness, which make them inappropriate for agitated depressed patients. They are very highly protein bound (90–95%) [33], meaning that they will complete with other highly bound medications such as digoxin, warfarin, and phenytoin. Thus, the free fraction of these medications will rise substantially, causing potential toxicity, while the blood levels (which measure total blood level, not just the free portion) will not reflect this. There is a small but significant incidence with fluoxetine of hyponatremia, which can mimic depression. Fluoxetine also has a 10% incidence of clinically significant weight loss, which is potentially troublesome in this population. Fluoxetine has a long half-life (approximately 2–3 days for the drug itself and 7–9 days for norfluoxetine, which is an active metabolite). The other SSRIs marketed at this time in the United States, sertraline and paroxetine, have much shorter half-lives of approximately 1 day [33]. Deaths have been reported when SSRIs were used in combination with monoamine oxidase inhibitors; note that the chemotherapeutic agent procarbazine has MAO inhibitor activity. A study is currently underway at Memorial Sloan-Kettering Cancer Center and several other centers [Lesko et al.] to prospectively compare the efficacy of fluoxetine with desipramine in late-stage cancer patients with depression.

Psychostimulants are very useful for patients with prominent symptoms of lethargy, cognitive slowing, and anergia. Used in terminal phases they can improve appetite, enhance self worth, and counter the sedative effects of narcotic pain mediations. They should be started at low doses (5 mg/day of dextroamphetamine or methylphenidate, or 37.5 mg/day of pemoline) and given a divided dose early morning and early afternoon to avoid excess nighttime stimulation. Pemoline has the disadvantage of occasional liver toxicity, requiring monitoring of liver enzymes during its use. It has the advantage of being available in a chewable preparation, which can be absorbed through the buccal mucosa even if patients are unable to swallow. This makes it extremely useful for patients such as those with severe mucositis from chemotherapy or radiation, who cannot take oral medications [34].

Confusional States

Confusional states are common in the cancer setting, both due to the direct involvement of the CNS by tumor and to the indirect effects on the CNS of the disease or its treatment. Although there is some controversy over how to make distinctions between delirium and other organic brain syndromes, in our center we tend to consider all acute mental status changes as having a similar treatment approach. The causes of confusional states in cancer patients may be classified as follows:

1 Direct effects
  a Primary brain tumors
  b Brain metastases from primary sites outside the CNS
2 Indirect effects
  a Infections (both CNS and non-CNS)
  b Metabolic problems
       Organ failure
       Electrolyte imbalances
  c Treatment effects
       Radiation
       Steroids
       Chemotherapeutic agents
       Other medications, such as analgesics or antibiotics
  d Nutrition
       Malnutrition due to chronic illness
  e Vascular complications
  f Remote effects
       Tumors that secrete psychoactive substances
       Paraneoplastic syndromes

The prevalence of delirium in cancer patients has ranged in various studies from 5 to 25%. These studies are summarized in table 3. Some of these studies report prevalence rates based on screening all hospital admissions, while others report the frequency of organic mental disorders among patients referred for psychiatric consultation. In addition, older age, preexisting dementia, and levels of physical disability are confounding factors that make it impossible to arrive at a uniform prevalence rate. At Memorial Sloan-Kettering Hospital, 15% of 546 patients seen by the psychiatric consultation service met the diagnostic criteria for delirium [35].

Early symptoms of delirium are often unrecognized or misdiagnosed as depression. Early recognition is important since the underlying etiology may be a treatable complication of cancer. When an abrupt change in behavior or cognition is recognized in a patient, a number of possible causes must be investigated. Particularly, frequent metabolic problems causing delirium include hyponatremia, hypercalcemia, malnutrition, and liver failure. Thyroid or adrenal status may be altered. Patients with hematologic malignancies or AIDS are at an especially high risk for opportunistic infections. Some cancers, such as those of the lung and breast, frequently metastasize to the brain. Because of these differences, the 'delirium workup' is not uniform for each patient but should be tailored to the patient's specific situation. Delirium as a side effect of chemotherapeutic agents is dealt with later in this chapter, in the section on the

Table 3. Twelve studies of delirium in hospitalized cancer patients

Reference	n	State or type of disease	Percentage with organic mental syndrome
Hospitalized patients (referred for psychiatric consultation)			
Hinton [10]	50	terminal illness	10
Shevitz et al. [36]	1,000	cancer and noncancer in a general hospital	16
Levine et al. [15]	100	all stages	40
Massie et al. [37]	334	all stages	25
Massie and Holland [20]	546	all stages	20
Hospitalized patients (not only those referred for psychiatric consultation)			
Davies [38]	46	advanced cancer	27
Posner [39]	–	CNS complications of cancer	15
Derogatis et al. [2]	215	all stages	8
Folstein [40]	83	consecutive admissions	26
Hospitalized patients on general medical and surgical services (cancer and noncancer patients)			
Lipowski [41]	–	general medical patients 'elderly'	16
Adams [42]	–	general surgical patients	10–15

Modified from Fleishman and Lesko [43].

specific side effects of these agents. Treatment is the same as the treatment for delirium arising from other causes.

Treatment of delirium is directed at ensuring the patient's safety, decreasing agitation and anxiety, improving orientation and cognition, and increasing comfort by minimizing dysphoria. The first line of management should be environmental manipulation. All unnecessary stimuli should be minimized, and a one-to-one companion may be needed, especially if the patient is disoriented, very agitated, or potentially violent. Patients who have worsening at night ('sundowning') may benefit from leaving a light and radio on at all times to help orient them. Physical restraints may be required if the patient is in imminent danger of hurting himself or others, either by physical violence or by leaving the hospital while severely ill. Care should be taken to avoid using restraints on patients who might be harmed by them due to their medical conditions, such as patients with thrombocytopenia or bone metastases.

The major medications used for the treatment of delirium and other acute confusional states in the cancer patient are the neuroleptics. Early use of these agents calms the patient to allow for easier workup of the possible etiology of the delirium, improves patient comfort, avoids prolonged use of physical restraints, and helps prevent progression to more florid states such as frank agitation or psychosis. The most commonly used pharmacologic agent for delirium is haloperidol, because of its low incidence of side effects such as sedation, cardiac toxicity, anticholinergic effects, and anti-α-adrenergic effects. In addition, it is available in a variety of forms (tablets, elixir, and parenteral). Although haloperidol is not FDA approved for intravenous administration, it is often used by this route for patients who are unable or unwilling to take it orally and when intramuscular administration is contraindicated because of conditions such as thrombocytopenia or the need for frequent dosing [44]. For acutely agitated patients at our center, haloperidol is given as 0.5–2.0 mg i.v. at the rate of 1 mg/min and repeated every 30 min until the patient is calm. If the agitation does not respond after several doses, or if the agitation is too severe to allow waiting for the effects of repeated haloperidol doses, then we add lorazepam 1–2 mg i.v. to the haloperidol dose. Patients are then maintained on a regimen of haloperidol, either orally or intravenously, that is equivalent to one-half to two-thirds of the dose required to calm the patient over the initial 24-hour period. To control agitation, most prefer this maintenance dose in a b.i.d. or t.i.d. regimen; a common method of administration is to give one-third of the dose in the morning and two-thirds at night.

Other clinicians have reported on other methods of using haloperidol, either alone or in combination with other medications, to control severe agitation. Adams [45] prefers to use a combination of haloperidol 5–10 mg i.v. push with lorazepam 0.5–2 mg i.v. push every 20–30 min, supplemented with hydromorphone 0.5 mg i.v. push every 3 h. While we have not found it necessary to use these doses to treat agitation, it is significant that high doses of both lorazepam and haloperidol have been found safe in delirious cancer patients. There is, however, one report of asystole induced by intravenous haloperidol [46].

For patients who do not have severe agitation, but do have prominent symptoms of anxiety and irritability, thioridazine may be very useful. However, its higher incidence of side effects (particularly anticholinergic, but also cardiotoxic, hepatotoxic, and sedative) should be remembered. In the low doses used for confusional states without severe agitation (see below), we have not found these to be problematic in cancer patients. Thioridazine is not available in a parenteral preparation, limiting its usefulness in acute situations with more severely agitated patients.

With patients who do not require immediate control of severe agitation, neuroleptics should be started at low dosages. For example, use 0.5–1.0 mg/day of haloperidol or 10–30 mg/day of thioridazine in elderly or debilitated patients, or 1.0–2.0 mg/day of haloperidol or 20–40 mg/day of thioridazine for patients in good physical condition. Increase the dose every 1–2 days by small amounts until clinical symptoms of agitation, confusion, and irritability are controlled. Since delirium is usually worse at night and is characterized by a reversed sleep-wake cycle, it is usually most helpful to give the major portion of the dose at night, but many patients benefit from having some medication in the morning or at midday as well.

Side effects of neuroleptic treatment should be monitored. The incidence of extrapyramidal symptoms (EPS) such as acute dystonia, parkinsonism, and akathisia is low with intravenous administration of neuroleptics [47]. EPS can be managed by reduction of the dose or by administration of low doses of anticholinergic agents such as 0.5–1.0 mg of benztropine per day. If agitation appears to worsen during haloperidol administration, the possibility of akathisia must be considered. Benzodiazepines can be a helpful adjunct to neuroleptics if this occurs. Neuroleptics also decrease the ability of the hypothalamus to regulate body temperature, so care should be taken to keep the temperature in a patient's room moderate. Finally, neuroleptic malignant syndrome is a very rare but potentially life-threatening complication of neuroleptic administration. It should be suspected in any patient who has more than one of the following: increasing confusion or agitation, increased temperature, other signs of autonomic disregulation, muscular rigidity, or increased blood levels of creatine phosphokinase. Treatment consists first of stopping the neuroleptic immediately, cooling and hydrating the patient, and if necessary administering bromocriptine or dantrolene [48].

Special Issues

Psychiatric Syndromes Related to Specific Cancer Treatments
Chemotherapy/Medication. Many of the chemotherapeutic agents used in the treatment of cancer have central nervous system toxicities. These are summarized in table 4. In addition to the standard antineoplastic drugs, biological response modifiers, antifungals, and antivirals have all been found to have CNS side effects. Recognition and management of these side effects leads to enhanced patient comfort and compliance with treatment.

Many chemotherapeutic agents do not cross the blood-brain barrier to any significant degree, and therefore produce few direct side effects on the central nervous system. Delirium is associated, however, with the use of methotrexate (especially with intrathecal or high-dose intravenous administration), 5-fluorouracil, the vinca alkaloids (vinblastine and vincristine), bleo-

Table 4. Chemotherapeutic agents and their CNS toxicities

	Delirium	Lethargy	Halluci-nations	Cognitive impairment	Depres-sion	EPS
5-Azacytidine				×		
Aminoglutethimide				×		
Asparaginase	×	×	×	×		
BCNU	×			×		
Bleomycin	×					
Cisplatinum	×					
Cytosine arabinoside	×	×		×		
Dacarbazine				×		
Fludarabine	×			×		
Fluorouracil	×					
Hydroxyurea			×			
Ifosfamide	×	×	×			
Methotrexate	×	×		×		×
Prednisone	×	×	×		×	
Procarbazine	×	×	×		×	
Vinblastine	×	×	×		×	
Vincristine	×	×	×			
Interferon	×	×	×			
Interleukin	×	×				

Modified from Lesko et al. [49].

mycin, carmustine (BCNU), cisplatin, *L*-asparaginase, procarbazine, Ara-C, ifosfamide and prednisone [49–54]. Cerebellar ataxia occurs infrequently from Ara-C, 5-fluorouracil, BNCU, and procarbazine. The vinca alkaloids, chemotherapeutic agents derived from the periwinkle plant and used in the treatment of leukemia and lymphoma, produce a peripheral neuropathy that can be severe and extremely painful for years after treatment is discontinued.

Corticosteroids are used in cancer treatment for several purposes: (1) to reduce cerebral edema associated with metastatic or primary brain tumor; (2) as a chemotherapeutic agent for leukemia and lymphoma; (3) combined with radiation to the spine when there are signs of cord compression, and (4) increasingly, as an adjunctive antiemetic agent in combination with metoclopramide, haloperidol, diphenhydramine, or lorazepam for chemotherapy protocols that utilize highly emetogenic drugs such as cisplatin. The initial psychologic response to steroids (euphoria and irritability) occur independently of the dose. Some effects are beneficial, providing a sense of well-being, increased appetite, and weight gain. Many effects, however, are uncomfortable, such as insomnia, restlessness, anxiety, hyperactivity, muscle weakness, fatigue, and depression. Severe effects are usually seen with higher doses but can be occur at small doses. Cessation of steroids can produce depression. Exaggerated responses to steroids, such as profound mood disturbance (mania or severe depression) or delirium, are less common. The drug-induced changes may be accompanied by hallucinations, paranoia, and delusions and are clinically indistinguishable from primary affective illness. These responses may appear when the dose is abruptly increased, tapered, or discontinued. Patients who require steroids as part of their chemotherapy, or who develop a spinal cord compression that demands emergency treatment, are given steroids even if they have a history of affective lability. Patient's moods should be carefully monitored, and pharmacologic treatment should be prescribed when necessary. Low doses of neuroleptics (0.5–3 mg of haloperidol or 10–40 mg of thioridazine per day) are used for initial treatment of steroid reactions, and the response to these can be dramatic. Other psychotropic agents should be avoided initially, since they can exacerbate confusion and agitation; however, if neuroleptics are ineffective, benzodiazepines (for anxiety and agitation) or antidepressants (for depression) may be added. As discussed previously, lithium has been found to be helpful in preventing steroid-induced affective changes in some patients; we usually reserve its use for manic states that are not fully responsive to neuroleptics. If steroid reactions occur during a rapid taper, the steroid dose should be increased and then lowered more gradually.

Biological response modifiers and immunotherapy agents represent promising new developments in cancer treatment. Neuropsychiatric disturbances have been reported with several immunological agents including interferon [55, 56] and interleukin-2 [57]. To date, the interferons have been used in clinical studies with hairy cell leukemia, chronic myelocytic leukemia and Kaposi's sarcoma. Intramuscular administration of interferon in dosages of 2–50 million units per day produces flu-like symptoms of lethargy, anorexia, headaches, nausea, or depression [58, 59]. A study of tumor necrosis factor in hepatitis B carriers in whom social class variables were controlled, using the General Health Questionnaire [60] found that interferon did increase psychiatric morbidity. The major symptoms were nonpsychotic ones, such as fatigue, poor concentration, anxiety, and depression. These side effects of interferon appear to be dose related and disappear upon discontinuation of the drug.

Amphotericin B is used regularly for the treatment of fungal infection in immunologically compromised cancer and AIDS patients. Because it is poorly absorbed via the gastrointestinal tract it is given intravenously. It can cause anaphylaxis, fever, rigors, anorexia, and impaired renal function. Various neurological side effects, including delirium, have been reported with intrathecal administration. Ellis et al. [61] reported 14 patients treated with the methyl ester of amphotericin B who developed progressive severe neurologic dysfunction including dementia, akathisia, mutism, hyperreflexia, tremor, and white-matter deterioration. Symptoms were dose dependent and were most severe with doses greater than 9.0 g. It is often difficult to distinguish CNS effects of antifungal medications from those of fever, CNS infections, or metabolic abnormalities.

Acyclovir is a relatively new antiviral drug that has proved efficacious for prophylaxis and treatment of herpes simplex and varicella zoster virus. It is widely used in patients who are immunologically compromised by AIDS, bone marrow transplantation, or leukemia. The use of parenteral acyclovir (750–3,000 mg/m^2/day) has been associated with minimal drug toxicity. Wade and Myers [62] reported reversible neurotoxicity in 6 of 143 bone marrow transplant recipients studies. Symptoms, which developed in a median of 8 days after the initiation of treatment, included lethargy in 5 patients, agitation in 5 patients, tremor in 5 patients, disorientation in 1 patient and transient hemiparasthesias in 1 patient. The authors noted that these patients may have been predisposed to neurologic side effects by previous intrathecal methotrexate therapy, total body irradiation, preexisting CNS leukemia, herpes virus infections, or the concurrent use of interferon. All patients improved with the discontinuation of acyclovir, suggesting that the transient CNS toxicity was secondary to the antiviral agent rather than to other factors.

Radiation Therapy. Whole brain radiation, used to treat primary as well as metastatic lesions of the brain, can be complicated by radiation-induced encephalopathy. Three types of encephalopathy have been described: (1) acute encephalopathy, seen immediately after the first radiation treatment; (2) early-delayed encephalopathy, beginning 6–16 weeks after treatment and (3) late-delayed encephalopathy, seen 6 months to several years later [63, 64].

An acute encephalopathy can occur during the immediate course of high-dose radiation therapy (RT). Patients can become lethargic, and complain of headache, nausea, vomiting, and fever. It is thought that this type of acute reaction is due to increased intracranial pressure secondary to radiation-induced changes in the blood-brain barrier. Left untreated it can lead to worsening of neurologic deficits and even brain herniation. Corticosteroids are the treatment of choice for this syndrome.

An 'early-delayed' encephalopathy usually begins 1–4 months after radiation treatment. Symptoms consist of lethargy, headache, nausea and vomiting. In children who receive whole brain RT prophylactically for leukemia, the picture is usually one of generalized somnolence and headache. Patients who receive more focal RT to the brain can present with symptoms of focal neurological disease suggestive or recurrence of tumor. The cause of early-delayed radiation encephalopathy is unknown, but may be related to radiation-induced edema or demyelination. Improvement in symptoms usually occurs spontaneously in 1–6 weeks. Steroids may be helpful in treating symptoms as well as for prophylaxis prior to or during RT.

A 'late-delayed' encephalopathy (usually severe and permanent) may develop 6 months to 3 years (average 12 months) after radiation therapy. This syndrome is characterized by symptoms that suggest a focal neurological lesion, accompanied by personality change and headache. Seizures can also complicate the picture. Differential diagnosis includes recurrent tumor, infarct, or abscess. A CT scan of the brain usually shows a hypodense lesion in the white matter. Biopsy of the brain will show necrosis. Clinically, radiation necrosis of the brain may present not only with symptoms of an organic mental disorder but also with personality changes and depression. The syndrome has been noted to resemble a subcortical dementia [65]. The depressive component of the syndrome has been reported to respond to antidepressant treatment despite the presence of underlying damage [66]. Steroids can help symptomatically; however, surgical resection of the necrotic mass is often necessary. Rowland et al. [67] found that children with acute lymphocytic leukemia who were treated with intrathecal methotrexate and cranial radiation as prophylaxis against CNS recurrence had a mean IQ 10 points lower than that of children who received only intrathecal methotrexate. Soft neurologic signs and abnormalities in growth hormone were also evident.

Nausea and Vomiting

Nausea and vomiting are frequent complications of cancer or its treatment. If untreated, vomiting may lead to dehydration, alterations in serum electrolytes, esophageal tears, malnutrition, or aspiration pneumonia. If nausea or vomiting are left untreated, patients may abandon conventional treatment or seek unproven alternative treatments.

The etiologies of nausea and vomiting are physiologic and metabolic, treatment-related, and psychological and behavioral. The first group of causes is relatively easy to identify but may be difficult to treat. It includes structural bowel obstruction due to tumor, metastases, or surgery; functional bowel obstruction due to mechanical or drug-related ileus; fluid and electrolyte imbalance; metabolic abnormalities such as ketoacidosis, uremia, and hepatic dysfunction; hypercalcemia, high fever; endocrine dysfunction such as adrenocortical insufficiency; and central nervous system dysfunction, such as primary brain tumor, metastatic disease, or increased intracranial pressure. Also causes of vomiting not related to cancer should not be overlooked, such as gastritis, ulcer, pancreatitis, renal or biliary colic, and myocardial infarction.

Nausea or vomiting is one of the most common side effects of cancer treatment. It may be produced by radiation, chemotherapeutic agents, narcotic analgesics, or intravenous antibiotics. Chemotherapy agents vary not only in their emetogenic potential but in their mechanism of producing nausea and vomiting. Cisplatin is highly emetogenic and causes vomiting by direct action on the vagus nerve, while 5-fluorouracil is mildly emetogenic and produces vomiting by directly stimulating the chemoreceptor trigger zone (CTZ). Table 5 shows the relative emetogenic potential of commonly used agents.

Behavioral and psychologic causes of nausea and vomiting are common in the cancer setting. Anticipatory nausea and vomiting follows a classical behavioral conditioning paradigm, in which anything inadvertently paired with the emetogenic stimulus (such as the sights and smells of the hospital or clinic) can later be sufficient to cause nausea or vomiting on its own. Current treatment consists of medications such as anxiolytics and antiemetics combined with behavioral techniques such as relaxation. A good reference for further information about anticipatory nausea and vomiting is the chapter by Redd [69].

Several classes of drugs have proven effective in the management of chemotherapy-induced nausea and vomiting. These include the dopamine antagonists (chlorpromazine, prochlorperazine, haloperidol, and metoclopramide) as well as adjunctive agents such as anticholinergics, antihistaminics, adrenergic stimulants such as dextroamphetamine, cannabinoids, benzodiazepines, and steroids.

Dopamine antagonists such as chlorpromazine, prochlorperazine, and haloperidol work by inhibiting dopamine activity at the CTZ. They are usually effective for patients receiving nitrosoureas or methotrexate, but are usually ineffective against the highly emetogenic agents such as cisplatin or doxorubicin. They can be administered parenterally, orally, or rectally (except for haloperidol which is not available in a rectal preparation). Since these drugs also block dopamine in other areas of the brain, patients can experience a variety of extrapyramidal symptoms such as dystonias, parkinsonism, or akathisia. These are treated with antihistamines (diphenhydramine) or anticholinergics (benztropine) just as with other patients who have these side effects. Once again, failure to treat these side effects aggressively can lead to patient frustration and noncompliance.

Metoclopramide is a procainamide derivative and also a CNS dopamine antagonist with peripheral gastrointestinal cholinergic effects. It was used initially in doses of 20–40 mg/day to increase lower esophageal tone, promote gastric emptying, and increase the motility of the upper gastrointestinal tract. More recently, it was found to be highly effective in controlling nausea and vomiting when used at high doses [70]. Given as 2 mg/kg i.v. 0.5 h prior to chemotherapy and repeated every 2 h for 2–5 doses, it was found to be more

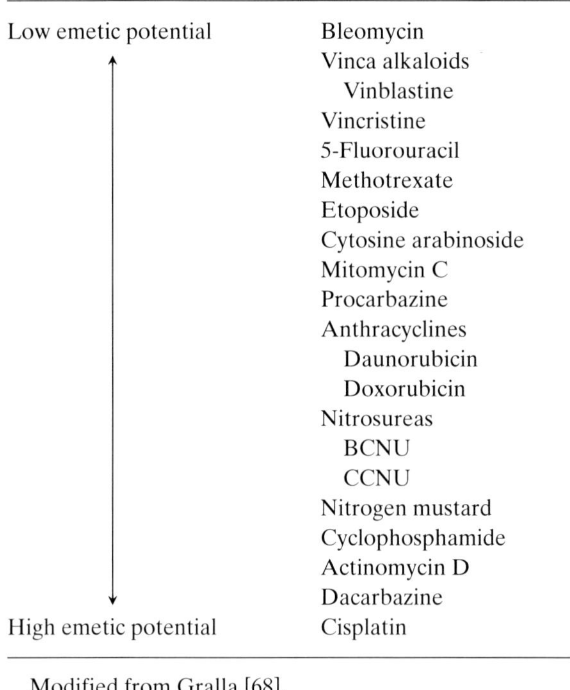

Table 5. Emetic potential of chemotherapy agents

Low emetic potential	Bleomycin
	Vinca alkaloids
	Vinblastine
	Vincristine
	5-Fluorouracil
	Methotrexate
	Etoposide
	Cytosine arabinoside
	Mitomycin C
	Procarbazine
	Anthracyclines
	Daunorubicin
	Doxorubicin
	Nitrosureas
	BCNU
	CCNU
	Nitrogen mustard
	Cyclophosphamide
	Actinomycin D
	Dacarbazine
High emetic potential	Cisplatin

Modified from Gralla [68].

effective for preventing emesis from cisplatin than either chlorpromazine (3.0 mg/kg) or haloperidol (1.0 mg/kg). The side effects of metoclopramide are similar to other dopamine antagonists, but are seen more frequently because of the high dosages used. Metoclopramide is usually given with diphenhydramine to alleviate this.

All of the dopamine antagonists can produce tardive dyskinesia with prolonged low-dose oral use [71, 72]; in addition, metoclopramide is capable of producing TD after short-term, high-dose parenteral use [73].

Cannabinoids such as delta-9-tetrahydrocannabinol (THC) and synthetic cannabinoids such as nabilone have been shown to have antiemetic activity for several chemotherapeutic agents, including high-dose methotrexate. It is felt that cannabinoids act centrally to raise the nausea and vomiting threshold of the emetic center. The average oral THC dose is 5–10 mg/m^2 (7.5–15 mg), given 2 h before chemotherapy and repeated every 3–4 h for 24–48 h. Side effects such as confusion and dysphoria are considerable for many patients, especially the elderly.

Agents that have been effective adjunctive antiemetics are anticholinergics, steroids and benzodiazepines. Anticholinergics (such as scopolamine) and antihistamines (such as diphenhydramine and hydroxyzine) are commonly used in labyrinthine-induced vomiting or motion sickness. They are inferior to the dopamine antagonists as sole agents in treatment of chemotherapy-induced emesis. Dexamethasone (3–20 mg, p.o. or i.v.) and methylprednisolone (200–500 mg i.v.) have some antiemetic activity. Parenteral lorazepam (2–5 mg i.v.) given prior to or concurrently with chemotherapy infusion may reduce vomiting and produces mild amnesia for vomiting episodes, thus lessening the development of anticipatory nausea and vomiting. The most effective regimens use a combination of medications (metoclopramide, steroids, lorazepam, and diphenhydramine), administered shortly before chemotherapy and continued up to 24–36 h after chemotherapy infusion is completed [74]. Most combined antiemetic regimens are designed for use with highly emetogenic chemotherapy protocols [75].

Recently, researchers have been exploring newer antiemetic agents with novel mechanisms of action. Ondansetron, a selective 5-HT$_3$ receptor antagonist, appears to be more effective than metoclopramide for prophylaxis of acute nausea and emesis secondary to cisplatin [76], especially in combination with dexamethasone [77]. These studies indicate the role of peripheral serotonin in mediating chemotherapy-induced nausea and vomiting. Besides its promising efficacy, ondansetron does not produce sedation, akathisia, or other extrapyramidal side effects. This side effect profile is especially attractive in treating the under-30 cancer population, where 25% of patients receiving metoclopramide develop extrapyramidal symptoms.

Anorexia

Anorexia, or loss of appetite, is one of the most common symptoms of cancer. Anorexia and the weight loss (cachexia) that accompanies it may be caused by the disease, by its treatment, or by psychological disorders. Medical cause include tumor, bowel obstruction, fever, reduced food intake, metabolic abnormalities (such as hepatic and renal dysfunction), infections, and ectopic hormone production by tumors. Loss of appetite develops because of surgery, radiation, and chemotherapy. Head and neck surgery may change facial architecture, limiting food intake, or alter oral and pharyngeal function, making chewing and swallowing difficult. Gastrectomy, pancreatectomy, and bowel resection may produce malabsorption and anorexia. Radiation produces acute side effects of glossitis, stomatitis, esophagitis, and altered sense of taste, all making it difficult to eat. Many of the chemotherapeutic agents, besides causing ulcerations of the gastrointestinal tract, produce nausea, vomiting and anorexia. Graft versus host disease, a serious complication of bone marrow transplantation, can cause diarrhea, abdominal pain, ileus, anorexia, weight loss, malabsorption, and failure to thrive. Antibiotics, antifungal agents, and pain medications produce anorexia. In general, cancer treatment alters the taste of food, the pleasure of eating, and the normal anatomic and metabolic processes.

Rare psychiatric syndromes and behavioral dynamics are often over-looked as the cause of appetite loss. Sometimes anorexia occurs in the context of depression or anxiety in the cancer patient. In such cases it may be difficult to determine cause and effect. Since cancer patients may not exhibit a full depressive syndrome, a trial of an antidepressant may be indicated if a patient has only a few of the symptoms of depression, such as poor sleep and appetite. Anorexia, in very rare instances, can emerge as a symptom of a previous psychiatric illness. Rare adolescents and young adults with eating disorders, such as anorexia nervosa and bulimia, bring to the cancer setting a complex set of preexisting psychological and behavioral dynamics. Learned food aversions, in which foods associated with nausea and vomiting are avoided, may also play a major role in cancer-related anorexia. Bernstein and colleagues [78], have demonstrated the phenomenon in pediatric cancer patients, but its clinical significance in patients with poor appetite is still unclear.

Several pharmacological agents are useful in promoting appetite and weight gain: antihistamines (cyproheptadine), steroids, cannabinoids, tricyclic antidepressants, and low doses of psychostimulants. Murphy [79] reports that dronabinol (THC), which is the active substance of marijuana and is used as an antiemetic, has also been shown to improve weight gain and reduce weight loss (by one pound per month). Appetite was increased by 50–75%. Megestrol acetate, a progestational drug used in women with breast cancer, promotes increased appetite and subsequent nonfluid weight gain in patients with both hormone-dependent and nonhormone-dependent tumors [80]. Sixteen percent of patients receiving 800 mg of megestrol acetate daily gained 15 lb or more over baseline within a 1- to 2-month period. A dose of 160–480 mg/day of megestrol acetate is more commonly used.

Patients with significant malnutrition who remain anorexic despite pharmacologic and environmental manipulations require formal nutritional support, such as enteral feedings via a nasogastric, gastrostomy, or jejunostomy tube, or total parenteral nutrition (TPN) via an indwelling central venous catheter. Untreated malnutrition can produce or exacerbate both mood disorders and delirium. Lesko [81] discusses the psychosocial issues of various types of enteral and parenteral feeding.

Management of anorexia can involve educational and behavioral as well as pharmacological approaches. Consultation from a nutritionist, involving family members at mealtimes, and decreasing anxiety with relaxation or self-hypnosis can all be useful in cancer patients for increasing intake. A patient's loss of anorexia and reversal of some cachexia frequently improves overall sense of well-being; its impact on cancer survival is unclear. Pharmacologic management of anorexia is more often used in terminally ill patients, however, whereas educational or behavioral techniques are used earlier in the course of illness and during active treatment.

Pain

In the PSYCOG study [2], each of the 215 patients rated the severity of their pain. Of patients who received a psychiatric diagnosis, 39% indicated the severity of their pain as being greater than 50 mm on a 100-mm visual analog scale. The most common psychiatric diagnoses of these patients were adjustment disorder with depressed or mixed mood (69%) or major depression (15%). By contrast, only 19% of patients who did not receive a psychiatric diagnosis had significant pain. This finding of increased frequency of psychiatric disturbance in patients with pain has been reported by others. Ahles et al. [82] compared cancer patients with pain and without pain, and found that patients with pain obtained higher scores on measures of depression, anxiety, hostility, and somatization. Sternbach [83] noted that anxiety symptoms often accompany acute pain, whereas depression is found in patients with chronic pain. Psychologic symptoms of anxiety or depression may be either a consequence of or a contributor to pain, and treating both usually has the effect of reducing pain.

The data just cited confirm clinical observations that psychiatric symptoms (e.g. anxiety, depression) of patients who are in pain must initially be considered as a consequence of uncontrolled pain. Acute anxiety, depression, despair (when the patient belives the pain means disease progression), anorexia, irritability, agitation, uncomfortableness, anger and change in sleep patterns are common emotional and behavioral symptoms of pain. Psychiatrists should first assist in the pharmacologic management of pain and then reassess the patient's mental state after pain is adequately controlled to determine whether the patient's symptoms are psychiatric in nature. In summary, the cancer patient with pain has an enhanced risk of developing psychiatric disorders commonly seen in cancer. Clearly, depression, anxiety, and mixed symptoms of depression and anxiety are the most common problems.

Pharmacologic therapy remains the mainstay of treatment of acute and chronic pain. The analgesic medications most commonly used are divided into these major categories [84]: (1) aspirin, acetaminophen, and nonsteroidal anti-inflammatory drugs, which peripherally produce analgesia via inhibition of the enzyme prostaglandin synthetase; (2) narcotic agonists and antagonists, which act centrally and peripherally by binding to opiate receptors and activating endogenous pain suppression, and (3) adjuvant drugs (antidepressants, antipsychotics) that act centrally to control pain by poorly understood mechanisms [85].

Foley [86] advocates an extensive assessment in a cancer patient with pain prior to attempting to treat that pain. Pain can be considered in 5 categories: (1) acute cancer-related pain secondary to disease or treatment (surgery, chemotherapy, radiation); (2) chronic pain related to tumor progression or treatment; (3) cancer-related pain and preexisting chronic pain; (4) cancer-related pain with history of drug addiction, and (5) pain in terminally ill patients.

Excellent guidelines for the pharmacologic management of pain are available [85, 86]. These principles include (1) treating the psychological as well as the physical symptoms of the pain; (2) using a specific drug for the specific pain (aspirin or nonsteroidal anti-inflammatory drugs are used for mild-to-moderate pain, and oral or parenteral narcotics for moderate to severe pain); (3) learning the pharmacology of the specific pain medication – analgesic dose for each route of administration, peak time and duration of analgesia, pharmacokinetics, and toxic side effects (e.g. sedation, respiratory depression, nausea, vomiting, constipation), administering analgesics regularly rather than on an 'as needed' basis; (5) being flexible in changing medications but allowing each analgesic an adequate trial; (6) watching for development of analgesic tolerance, physical dependence, and withdrawal; (7) not using placebos; (8) considering the use of combinations of drugs to enhance analgesia (e.g. narcotic analgesic with non-narcotic analgesic, dextroamphetamine, hydroxyzine, or amitriptyline) [87], and (9) adequately managing pain in terminal illness by morphine infusion [88].

The principles of using tricyclic antidepressants as adjuncts for cancer pain control are similar to those employed when they are used for depression. As discussed above, these include starting with a low dose such as 10–25 mg of amitriptyline or imipramine, raising the dose slowly, and monitoring carefully for side effects. Blood levels can be helpful in making dosage adjustments. Dosages and blood levels needed to achieve analgesic effects are similar to those needed for antidepressant effect [89]. Psychostimulants are useful in combination with narcotic analgesics, both to enhance pain relief and to diminish excess sedation [90]. Once again, the doses used for this purpose are similar to those used for treatment of depression in the oncology population.

Advanced AIDS

Recognition and treatment of advanced HIV-related psychiatric problems is becoming important as the incidence of infection increases and better supportive care emerges. HIV can directly affect the CNS, causing the 'AIDS dementia complex', or mental status changes can be due to opportunistic CNS infections such as toxoplasmosis and cryptococcal meningitis or tumors such as CNS lymphoma. Patients with advanced HIV are also vulnerable to the full spectrum of organic mental disorders, due to metabolic abnormalities, sepsis, medications, hypoxia, anemia, or malnutrition. Treatments for HIV may also cause organic mental syndromes. Zidovudine (AZT) has been reported to cause irritability and mania [91]. Interferon and other immune modulators are used in the treatment of Kaposi's sarcoma; the psychiatric complications of these drugs were discussed above, in the section on side effects of specific medications.

Eighty to ninety percent of autopsied AIDS patients have the histopathological changes in their brain tissue (microglial nodules and giant cell encephalitis) which are associated with HIV infection [92]. HIV involvement of the brain was initially described as dementia [93]; hence, the name AIDS dementia complex. However, Perry and Jacobsen [94] have reported that HIV infection can also present as delirium, psychosis, or depression; other case reports indicate that it can present with mania [95–97]. The prevalence in late HIV infection of such AIDS-related organic mental disorders which mimic functional psychiatric conditions is not known.

Treatment of advance HIV-related psychiatric conditions is dependent on both the specific symptoms and their cause. Correction of treatable etiologies such as electrolyte abnormalities, hypoxia, and infections should occur first. Patients with an altered mental status of any sort should have a head-imaging procedure (CT or MRI) and a lumbar puncture to rule out causes such as CNS lymphoma, mass lesions such as those due to toxoplasmosis, or infections such as neurosyphilis or cryptococcal meningitis. Suicide should be carefully assessed in patients with advanced HIV, since several studies indicate that suicide rates of men with AIDS was 20- to 35-fold higher than men without AIDS [98, 99]. Whether this is due to organic mental disorders, premorbid psychiatric disorders, substance abuse, or psychosocial stressors is not known. For patients with depression, psychostimulants have been shown to be efficacious for apathy, lethargy and withdrawal [100]. Other antidepressants can and should be employed, provided that low dosages are used and blood levels are monitored (if available for the agent used) to prevent excessive side effects.

Administration of high-potency neuroleptics to patients with AIDS-related delirium and psychosis has been associated with more frequent dystonic reactions and neuroleptic malignant syndrome [101–103]. This suggests that patients with advanced AIDS should be treated with low-potency neuroleptics. However, a study by Breitbart et al. [104] suggests that the dose used may be more important than the potency of the agent. This study found that low doses of neuroleptics, whether high potency or low potency, were effective in treating delirium. They were also safe, with no clinically significant side effects noted in the dosages used (0.5–2.0 mg haloperidol per day or 40–80 mg chlorpromazine per day).

A study at our center [105] has found that 38% of patients in an ambulatory outpatient AIDS clinic had significant pain. Furthermore, patients with pain had significantly more depression and functional impairment than patients without pain. This suggests that pain in the setting of AIDS should be assessed and treated as it is in cancer patients (see the section on 'Pain', above).

Summary and Conclusions

This chapter has reviewed the prevalence of cancer and of psychiatric syndromes in the cancer setting. Guidelines have been given for the evaluation and treatment of specific psychiatric syndromes, as well as several special problems found in the cancer setting. In general, the major principle of using psychiatric medications in the patient with cancer or advanced AIDS is to use them to improve comfort, and not to withhold them when they may be of benefit.

References

1   DeVita VT, Oliverio VT, Muggia FM, Wiernik PW, Zeigler J, Goldin A, Rudin D, Henney J, Schepartz S: The drug development and clinical trials programs of the Division of Cancer Treatment, National Cancer Institute. Cancer Clin Trials 1979;2:195–216.
2   Derogatis LR, Morrow GR, Fetting J, Penman D, Piatsetsky MA, Schmale AM, Henricks M, Carnicke CLM: The prevalence of psychiatric disorders among cancer patients. JAMA 1983; 249:751–757.
3   Busto U, Sellers EM, Naranjo CA, Cappell H, Sanchez-Craig M, Sykora K: Withdrawal reaction after long-term use of benzodiazepines. N Engl J Med 1986;315:854–859.
4   Dominguez RA, Goldstein BJ: 25 years of benzodiazepine experience: Clinical commentary on use, abuse, and withdrawal. Hosp Formul 1985;20:1000–1014.
5   Massie MJ, Lesko L: Psychopharmacological management; in Holland JC, Rowland JH (eds): Handbook of Psychooncology. New York, Oxford University Press, 1989, pp 470–491.
6   Jenike M: Treating anxiety in elderly patients. Geriatrics 1983;38:115–119.
7   Massie MJ, Holland JC, Straker N: Psychotherapeutic interventions; in Holland JC, Rowland JH (eds): Handbook of Psychooncology. New York, Oxford University Press, 1989, pp 455–469.
8   Mastrovito R: Behavioral techniques: Progressive, relation, and self-regulatory therapies; in Holland JC, Rowland JH (eds): Handbook of Psychooncology. New York, Oxford University Press, 1989, pp 492–501.
9   Lansky SB, List MA, Herrman CA, Ets-Hokin EG, DasGupta TK, Wilbanks GD, Hendrickson FR: Absence of major depressive disorder in female cancer patients. J Clin Oncol 1985; 3:1553–1560.
10 Hinton J: Psychiatric consultation in fatal illness. Proc R Soc Med 1972;65:1035–1038.
11 Koenig R, Levin SF, Brennan MJ: The emotional status of cancer patient as measured by a psychological test. J Chron Dis 1967;20:923–30.
12 Peck A, Boland L: Emotional reaction to having cancer. Am J Roentgenol Radiat Ther Nucl Med 1972;114:591–599.

13   Craig TJ, Abeloff MD: Psychiatric symptomatology among hospitalized cancer patients. Am J Psychiatry 1974;131:1323–1327.

14   Plumb MM, Holland JC: Comparative studies of psychological function in patients with advanced cancer. I. Self-reported depressive symptoms. Psychosom Med 1977;39:264–276.

15   Levine PM, Silberfarb PM, Lipowski ZJ: Mental disorders in cancer patients: A study of 100 psychiatric referrals. Cancer 1978;42:1385–1391.

16   Massie MJ, Gorzynski JG, Mastrovito R, Theis D, Holland JC: The diagnosis of depression in hospitalized patients with cancer. Proc Am Soc Clin Oncol 1979;20:432.

17   Plumb MM, Holland JC: Comparative studies of psychological function in patients with advanced cancer. II. Interviewer-rated current and past psychological symptoms. Psychosom Med 1981;43:243–254.

18   Bukberg J, Penman D, Holland JC: Depression in hospitalized cancer patients. Psychosom Med 1984;46:199–212.

19   Evans DL, McCartney CF, Nemeroff CB, Raft D, Quade D, Golden RN, Haggerty JJ, Holmes V, Simons JS, Droba M, Mason GA, Fowler WC: Depression in women treated for gynecological cancer: Clinical and neuroendocrine assessment. Am J Psychiatry 1986;143:447–452.

20   Massie MJ, Holland JC: The cancer patient with pain: Psychiatric complications and their management. Med Clin North Am 1987;71:243–258.

21   Massie MJ: Depression; in Holland JC, Rowland JH (eds): Handbook of Psychooncology. New York, Oxford University Press, 1989, pp 284–286.

22   Purohit D, Navlakha P, Modi S, Eshpumiyami R: The role of antidepressants in hospitalized cancer patients. J Assoc Physns India 1978;26:245–248.

23   Costa D, Mogos I, Toma T: Efficacy and safety of mianserin in the treatment of depression of women with breast cancer. Acta Psychiatr Scand 1985;72:85–92.

24   Maguire P, Hopwood P, Tarrier N, Howell T: Treatment of depression in cancer patients. Acta Psychiatr Scand 1985;72:81–84.

25   Lansky S: Only a small number of clinically depressed cancer patients can be managed by drugs. Clin Psychiatry News, March 25, 1987, p 25.

26   Holland JC, Morrow GR, Schmale A, Derogatis LR, Stefanek M, Berenson S, Carpenter PJ, Breitbart W, Feldstein M: A randomized clinical trial of alprazolam versus progressive muscle relaxation in cancer patients with anxiety and depressive symptoms. J Clin Oncol 1991;9:1–8.

27   Evans DL, McCartney CF, Haggerty JJ, Nemeroff CB, Golden RN, Simon JB, Quade D,- Holmes V, Droba M, Mason GA, Fowler WC, Raft D: Treatment of depression in cancer patients is associated with better life adaptation: A pilot study. Psychosom Med 1988;50:72–76.

28   Carroll B: Alprazolam, promising in the treatment of depression in cancer patients. Psychiatr Times May 1990:46–47.

29   Mermelstein H, Lesko L: Depression in patients with cancer. Psychooncology 1992;1:207.

30   Speigel K, Kalb R, Pasternak GW. Analgesic activity of tricyclic antidepressants. Ann Neurol 1983;13:462–465.

31   Goggans FC, Wishberg LJ, Koran LM: Lithium prophylaxis of prednisone psychosis: A case report. J Clin Psychiatry 1983;44:111–112.

32   Scala SM, Visconti JA: Lithium in the treatment of leukemia. Hosp Form 1985;20:613–628.

33   DeVane CL: Pharmacokinetics of the selective serotonin reuptake inhibitors. J Clin Psychiatry 1992;53(suppl):13–20.

34   Breitbart W, Mermelstein H: Pemoline: An alternative psychostimulant for the management of depressive disorders in cancer patients. Psychosomatics 1992;33:352–356.

35   Massie MJ, Holland JC: Psychiatry and oncology; in Grinspoon L (ed): Psychiatry Update, vol III. Washington, American Psychiatric Press, 1984, pp 239–256.

36   Shevitz SA, Silberfarb PM, Lipowski ZJ: Psychiatric consultations in a general hospital: A report of 1000 referrals. Dis Nerv Syst 1976;37:295–300.

37   Massie MJ, Holland JC, Glass E: Delirium in terminally ill cancer patients. Am J Psychiatry 1983;140:1048–1050.

38   Davies RK, Quinlan DM, McKegney FP, Kimball CP: Organic factors and psychological adjustment in advanced cancer patients. Psychosom Med 1973;35:464–471.

39   Posner JB: Delirium and exogenous metabolic brain disease; in Beeson PB, McDermott WM, Wyngaarden (eds): Cecil Textbook of Medicine. Philadelphia, Saunders, 1979, pp 644–651.

40   Folstein MF, Fetting JH, Lobo A, Niaz U, Capozzoli K: Cognitive assessment of cancer patients. Cancer 1984;53(suppl May 15):2250–2255.

41   Lipowski ZJ: Transient cognitive disorders (delirium, acute confusional states) in the elderly. Am J Psychiatry 1983;140:1426–1436.

42   Adams F: Neuropsychiatric evaluation and treatment of delirium in the critically ill cancer patient. Cancer Bull Univ Texas M.D. Anderson Hosp Tumor Inst 1984;36:156–160.

43   Fleishman SB, Lesko LM: Delirium and dementia; in Holland J, Rowland JH (eds): Handbook of Psychooncology. New York, Oxford University Press, 1989, p 345.

44   Dudley DL, Rowlett DE, Loebel PJ: Emergency use of intravenous haloperidol. Gen Hosp Psychiatry 1979;1:240–246.

45   Adams F: Emergency intravenous sedation of the delirious, medically ill patient. J Clin Psychiatry 1988;49(suppl):22–27.

46   Huyse F, Van Schijndel RS: Haloperidol and cardiac arrest. Lancet 1988;ii:568–569.

47   Menza MA, Murray GB, Holmes VF, Rafuls WA: Decreased extrapyramidal symptoms with the use of intravenous haloperidol. J Clin Psychiatry 1987;48:178–280.

48   Guze BH, Baxter LR: Neuroleptic malignant syndrome. N Engl J Med 1985;313:163–166.

49   Lesko LM, Massie MJ, Holland JC: Oncology; in Stoudemire A, Fogel BS (eds): Principles of Medical Psychiatry, ed 2. Orlando, Grune & Stratton, 1993, pp 565–590.

50   Young DF, Posner JB: Nervous system toxicity of the chemotherapeutic agents; in Vinken PJ, Bruyn GW (eds): Neurological Manifestations of Systemic Diseases. II. Handbook of Clinical Neurology. New York, Elsevier Biomedical Press, 1980, vol 39, pp 91–129.

51   Kaplan RS, Wiernik PH: Neurotoxicity of antineoplastic drugs. Semin Oncol 1983;9:103–130.

52   Zapluski M, Baker LH: Ifosfamide. J Natl Cancer Inst 1988;80:556–566.

53   Fleishman SB, Lesko LM: Delirium and dementia; in Holland JC, Rowland JH (eds): Handbook of Psychooncology. New York, Oxford University Press, 1989, pp 342–355.

54   Moore DH, Fowler WC, Crumpler LS: Fluorouracil neurotoxicity. Gynecol Oncol 1990;36:152–154.

55   Adams F, Quesada JR, Gutterman JU: Neuropsychiatric manifestations of human leukocyte interferon therapy in patients with cancer. JAMA 1984;252:938–941.

56   Quesada JR, Talpaz M, Rios A, Kurzrock R, Gutterman JU: Clinical toxicity of interferons in cancer patients: A review. J Clin Oncol 1986;4:234–243.

57   Denicoff KD, Rubinoff DR, Pappa MZ, Simpson C, Seipp CA, Lotze MT, Chung AE, Rosenstein D, Rosenberg SA: The neuropsychiatric effects of treatment with interleukin-2 and lymphokine-activated killer cells. Ann Intern Med 1987;107:293–300.

58   Rohatiner AZS, Prior PF, Burton AC, Smith AT, Balkwill FR, Lister TA: Central nervous system toxicity of interferon. Br J Cancer 1983;47:419–442.

59   Smedley H, Katrak M, Sikora K, Wheeler T: Neurologic effects of recombinant human interferon. Br Med J 1983;286:262–264.

60   McDonald EM, Mann AH, Thomas HC: Interferons as mediators of psychiatric morbidity: An investigation in the trial of recombinant alpha interferon in hepatitis-B carriers. Lancet 1987;ii:1175–1178.

61   Ellis WG, Sobel RA, Nielsen SL: Leukoencephalopathy in patients treated with amphotericin B methyl ester. J Infect Dis 1982;126:125–137.

62   Wade JC, Myers JD: Neurological symptoms associated with parenteral acyclovir treatment after marrow transplantation. Ann Intern Med 1983;98:921–925.

63   Sheline GE: Irradiation injury of the human brain: A review of clinical experience; in Gilbert J, Kagan AR (eds): Radiation Damage to the Nervous System. New York, Raven Press, 1980, pp 39–58.

64   Patchell RA, Posner JB: Cancer and the nervous system; in Holland JC, Rowland JH (eds): Handbook of Psychooncology. New York, Oxford University Press, 1989, pp 327–341.

65   DeAngelis LM, Delattre J, Posner JB: Radiation-induced dementia in patients cured of brain metastases. Neurology 1989;39:789–796.

66   McMahon T, Vahora S: Radiation damage to the brain: Neuropsychiatric aspects. Gen Hosp Psychiatry 1986;8:437–441.

67   Rowland JH, Glidwell OJ, Sobley RF, Holland JC, Tull R, Berman A, Brecher ML, Harris M, Glicksman AS, Forman E, Jones B, Cohen ME, Duffer PK, Freemen AI: Effects of different forms of central nervous system prophylaxis and neuropsychologic function in childhood leukemia. J Clin Oncol 1984;2:1327–1335.

68   Gralla RJ: The control of nausea and vomiting in patients; in Bosl (ed): Current Concepts in Medical Oncology 1985. New York, Memorial Sloan-Kettering Cancer Center, 1985, p 50.

69   Redd WH: Management of anticipatory nausea and vomiting; in Holland JC, Rowland JH (eds): Handbook of Psychooncology. New York, Oxford University Press, 1989, pp 423–433.

70   Gralla JR, Itri LM, Pisko SE, Squillante AE, Kelsen DP, Braun DW, Bordin LA, Braun TJ, Young CW: Antiemetic efficacy of high dose metoclopramide: Randomized trials with placebo and prochlorperazine in patients with chemotherapy-induced nausea and vomiting. N Engl J Med 1981;305:905–909.

71   Lazzara RR, Stoudemire A, Manning D, Prewitt KC: Metoclopramide induced tardive dyskinesia: A case report. Gen Hosp Psychiatry 1986;8:107–109.

72   Wilholm B-E, Mortimer O, Boethius G, Haggstrom JE: Tardive dyskinesia associated with metoclopramide. Br Med J 1984;288:545–547.

73   Breitbart W: Tardive dyskinesia associated with high dose intravenous metoclopramide. N Engl J Med 1986;315:518.

74   Gralla RJ: Antiemetic therapy and cancer chemotherapy; in Hellman K, Carter SK (eds): Fundamentals of Cancer Chemotherapy. New York, McGraw-Hill, 1987, pp 387–396.

75   Strum SF, McDermed JE, Steng BR, McDermott NM: Combination metoclopramide and dexamethasone: An effective antiemetic regimen in outpatients receiving non-cisplatin chemotherapy. J Clin Oncol 1984;2:1057–1063.

76   Marty M, Pouillart P, Scholl S, Droz JP, Azab M, Brion N, Pujade-Lauraine E, Paule B, Paes D, Bons J: Comparison of the 5-hydroxy tryptamine (serotonin) antagonist ondansetron (GR 38032F) with high-dose metoclopramide in the control of cisplatin-induced emesis. N Engl J Med 1990;322:816–821.

77   Smith DB, Newlands ES, Rustin GJS, Begent RHJ, Howells N, McQuade B, Bagshawe KD: Comparison of ondansetron and ondansetron plus dexamethasone as antiemetic prophylaxis during cisplatin-containing chemotherapy. Lancet 1991;338:487–490.

78   Bernstein Il: Etiology of anorexia in cancer. Cancer 1986;58:1881–1886.

79   Murphy G: American Cancer Society Medical Affairs Newsletter II. 1990;ii:B.

80   Feliu J, Gonzalez-Baron M, Berrocal A, Artal A, Ordonez A, Garrido P, Zamora P, Garcia de Paredes ML, Montero JM: Usefulness of megestrol acetate in cancer cachexia and anorexia. Am J Clin Oncol 1992;15:436–440.

81   Lesko LM: Anorexia; in Holland JC, Rowland JH (eds): Handbook of Psychooncology. New York, Oxford University Press, 1989, pp 434–443.

82   Ahles TA, Blanchard EB, Ruckdeschel JC: Multidimensional nature of cancer-related pain. Pain 1983;17:227–228.

83   Sternbach RA: Pain Patients: Treats and Treatment. New York, Academic Press, 1974.

84   Moulin DE, Foley KM: Management of pain in patients with cancer. Psychiatr Ann 1984;14:815–822.

85   Foley KM: Pharmacologic management of pain; in Massie MJ, Lesko LM (eds): Current Concepts in Psychooncology. New York, Gold Publishers, 1984, pp 29–32.

86   Foley KM: Non-narcotic and narcotic analgesics: Applications; in Foley KM (ed): Management of Cancer Pain. New York, Gold Publishers, 1986, pp 135–152.

87   Walsh TD: Controlled study of imipramine and morphine in chronic pain due to advanced cancer. Proc Am Soc Clin Oncol 1986;5:237.

88   Portenoy RK, Moulin DF, Roger A, Inturrisi CE, Foley KM: Intravenous infusion of opioids in cancer pain: Clinical review and guidelines for use. Cancer Treat Rep 1986;70:575–581.

89 Max MB, Culnane M, Schafer SC, Gracely RH, Walther DJ, Smoller B, Dubner R: Amitriptyline relieves diabetic neuropathy pain in patients with normal and depressed mood. Neurology 1987;37:589–596.
90 Bruera E, Brenneis C, Paterson AH, MacDonald RN: Use of methylphenidate as an adjuvant to narcotic analgesics in patients with advanced cancer. J Pain Sympt Management 1989;4: 3–6.
91 Maxwell S, Scheftner WA, Kessler HA, Busch K: Manic syndrome associated with zidovudine treatment. JAMA 1988;259:3406–3407.
92 Navia BA, Cho ES, Rosenblum ML: The AIDS dementia complex. II. Neuropathology. Ann Neurol 1986;19:525–535.
93 Navia BA, Price RW: The acquired immunodeficiency syndrome dementia complex as the presenting or sole manifestation of human immunodeficiency virus infection. Arch Neurol 1987; 44:65–69.
94 Perry SW, Jacobsen P: Neuropsychiatric manifestations of AIDS-spectrum disorders. Hosp Community Psychiatry 1986;37:135–143.
95 Kermani EJ, Borod JC, Brown PH, Tunnell G: New psychopathologic findings in AIDS: Case report. J Clin Psychiatry 1985;46:240–241.
96 Schmidt U, Miller D: Two cases of hypomania in AIDS. Br J Psychiatry 1988;152:839–842.
97 Boccellari A, Dilley JW, Shore MD: Neuropsychiatric aspects of AIDS dementia complex: A report on a clinical series. Neurotoxicology 1988;9:381–389.
98 Marzuk PM, Tierney H, Tardiff K, Gross EM, Morgan EB, Hsu M-A, Mann JJ: Increased risk of suicide in patients with AIDS. JAMA 1988;259:1333–1337.
99 Kizer KW, Green M, Perkins CI, Doebbert G, Hughes MJ: AIDS and suicide in California (letter). JAMA 1988;260:1881.
100 Holmes VF, Fernandez F, Levy JK: Psychostimulant in AIDS-related complex patients. J Clin Psychiatry 1989;50:5–8.
101 Edelstein J, Knight RT: Severe parkinsonism in two AIDS patients taking prochlorperazine (letter). Lancet 1987;ii:341–342.
102 Breitbart W, Marotta R, Call P: AIDS and neuroleptic malignant syndrome (letter). Lancet 1988;ii:1488–1489.
103 Swenson JR, Erman M, Labelle J, Demsdale JE: Extrapyramidal reactions: Neuropsychiatric mimics in patients with AIDS. Gen Hosp Psychiatry 1989;11:248–253.
104 Breitbart W, Platt M, Marotta R, Cobrera K, Gran C, Raymond S, Weisman K, Derevenco M: Low dose neuroleptic treatment for AIDS delirium (poster). Am Psychiatr Assoc 144th Ann Meet 1991.
105 Breitbart W, Passik S, Bronaugh T, Zale C, Bluestine S, Gomez M, Galer B, Portenoy R: Pain in the ambulatory AIDS patient: Prevalence and psychosocial correlates (abstract). 38th Ann Meet Acad Psychosomatic Med, October 17–20, 1991.

Steven Bluestine, MD, Psychiatry, Memorial Sloan-Kettering Cancer Center,
New York, NY 10021 (USA)

Silver PA (ed): Psychotropic Drug Use in the Medically Ill.
Adv Psychosom Med. Basel, Karger, 1994, vol 21, pp 138–162

Treatment of Mania in the Medically Ill

Krishna DasGupta[a], *James W. Jefferson*[b]

[a] Citadel Psychiatric Clinic, Fort Wayne, Ind.;
[b] Dean Foundation for Health, Research and Education, Madison, Wisc., USA

Many patients who require treatment for mania suffer from concurrent medical illnesses. While antimanic agents are not contraindicated in such patients, knowledge of potential adverse effects which may exacerbate medical illness is essential. In addition, the potential for adverse drug interactions must be considered. Treatment of such patients requires active and careful collaboration between psychiatrists and nonpsychiatric physicians.

Treatment of Mania

This chapter will focus on the use of lithium, carbamazepine, and valproate in the treatment of mania in patients with coexisting medical illness. Important drug interactions are reviewed in regard to each organ system. Because all possible drug interactions cannot be covered in this review, clinicians are encouraged to consult an appropriate publication or regional drug information center for further information. Antipsychotics and benzodiazepines, often used acutely in the treatment of mania, will not be addressed in this chapter. In addition, other drugs less firmly established as effective antimanic agents such as calcium channel blockers, fenfluramine, clonidine, and others, will not be discussed. In retrospective studies and a prospective comparison with lithium, electroconvulsive therapy (ECT) has been demonstrated to be an effective treatment for mania [1, 2]. Because of its rapid onset of action, ECT may be especially useful in severely manic patients with marked psychomotor agitation or dehydration. The comparative efficacy and safety of ECT versus medication in the medically ill manic patient has never been studied. Intuitively, one might expect ECT to be preferred because it is a brief and closely monitored treatment. Treatment decisions must be based on clinical experience, type of medical illness and how it might be altered by the various therapeutic modalities available.

Before treating mania in a medically ill patient, a clinician must be sure that the patient is not suffering from an organic mood disorder (secondary mania) caused by medical illness or medication. Illnesses known to be associated with mania include tumors, cerebrovascular disease, multiple sclerosis, hyperthyroidism, and others. Drugs, such as *l*-dopa, bromocriptine, corticosteroids, and others have also been shown in induce mania.

Lithium is the only drug with Food and Drug Administration (FDA) approval for treatment of acute mania and prevention of future episodes in bipolar patients. Lithium's effectiveness in the treatment of mania has been established in comparison with placebo, antipsychotics, and anticonvulsants.

Carbamazepine is currently the best studied alternative to lithium. There are now at least 13 double-blind, controlled trials comparing carbamazepine with placebo, lithium, and antipsychotics [2]. Carbamazepine appears to be an effective agent in the treatment of mania, and a favorable response occurs in approximately 60%. Because many carbamazepine studies involved treatment-resistant patients, direct comparisons of efficacy between lithium and carbamazepine are limited.

In recent years, valproate has generated increasing research interest as a potentially effective mood-stabilizing agent. Recent double-blind studies suggest valproate is effective in the treatment of mania [1, 3a]. A large multicenter inpatient study was recently completed showing valproate and lithium to be equally effective in treating acute mania [3b] a new drug application (NDA) was recently filed with the FDA for this indication.

Treatment of Mania in the Presence of Thyroid Disease

Lithium

Several authors have reported development of goiter in lithium-treated patients at a rate of approximately 4% per year [4–7]. Others have found either no goiter development [8–10] or a substantially higher prevalence [11–13]. Most report that lithium discontinuation and/or treatment with thyroid hormone will lead to goiter shrinkage over 1–3 months.

Most series have reported a 2–15% prevalence of lithium-induced hypothyroidism [14]. Although some state that most lithium-treated patients who become hypothyroid have preexisting autoimmune thyroiditis, others have found half to be antibody negative [15, 16]. Other investigators have reported early and transient laboratory evidence of hypothyroidism (decreased T4 and elevated TSH without clinical manifestations) that normalized with continued lithium treatment [16, 17a, b]. When patients with preexisting hypothyroidism require lithium, one must carry out a thorough evaluation which includes a physical examination, T4, TSH, and antithyroid (antithyroglobulin and antimicrosomal) antibody titers followed by adequate thyroid replacement. It is not known whether administration of lithium to patients with adequately treated preexisting hypothyroidism generally aggravates the condition, but it would be prudent to assume this to be the case. In addition to evaluating thyroid function when symptoms appear, we would suggest periodic thyroid function evaluation (T4, sensitive TSH) with appropriate dose adjustment of exogenous thyroid hormone. We also recommend regular monitoring of antithyroid antibody titers in those with baseline elevated titers, since such patients appear to be at increased risk for lithium-induced hypothyroidism.

Increased thyroid activity and thyrotoxicosis related to lithium treatment have rarely been reported [14, 18]; however, a few investigators have described patients who developed hyperthyroidism within several months of lithium discontinuation [19, 20]. If patients with preexisting hyperthyroidism require lithium for treatment of mania, we recommend thorough thyroid function evaluation before starting lithium to ensure hyperthyroidism has been appropriately treated. Whether patients with preexisting hyperthyroidism are at increased risk for lithium-induced hypo- or hyperthyroidism is not known. Because of its thyroid suppressant effect, lithium has been used investigationally to treat hyperthyroidism [21–24]. We recommend periodic evaluation of thyroid function in this potentially high-risk group.

Carbamazepine
Carbamazepine is associated with statistically significant decreases in serum T3 and T4, but serum TSH does not usually increase [25a, b]. Hormone levels decrease after 1–5 months of carbamazepine treatment. In one study, the frequency of clinically detectable goiter was significantly higher in carbamazepine-treated patients when compared with controls [26]. Whether those with preexisting thyroid disease are at increased risk for carbamazepine-induced hypothyroidism is not known. In addition, whether the rate of hypothyroidism is greater in patients treated concurrently with carbamazepine and lithium than in those treated with either agent alone has not been investigated. We recommend careful evaluation of baseline thyroid function with regular reassessment during carbamazepine treatment in these potentially high-risk groups.

Valproate

Dose-related decreases in T4 and T3 without changes in TSH have been described in valproate-treated patients [27]. Whether those with preexisting thyroid disease are at increased risk for valproate-induced hypothyroidism is not known, but we would recommend baseline and routine thyroid function evaluation as described above for patients with preexisting thyroid disease treated with lithium or carbamazepine.

Treatment of Mania in the Presence of Renal Disease

Lithium

Polyuria is a common side effect of lithium which may occur shortly after starting lithium or after many years of treatment. The incidence of polyuria is estimated to be between 2 and 35% [28]. Although maintaining patients at lower serum lithium levels is associated with less polyuria, a recent study suggests lower maintenance serum lithium levels may be associated with an increased relapse rate [29]. Although polyuria was initially considered a purely functional and reversible defect, studies suggest lithium may cause irreversible structural tubular damage leading to permanent changes in concentrating capacity and urine volume [30–33].

Morphological kidney changes occur in under 15% of unselected lithium-treated patients [28]. Lesions found include interstitial fibrosis, tubular atrophy, and glomerular sclerosis. In addition, a unique distal nephron lesion characterized by cytoplasmic swelling, accumulation of glycogen deposits, dilated tubules, and microcyst formation has been described in lithium-treated patients, but not psychiatric controls [34, 15a, b]. While some conclude this unique tubular lesion may lead to focal nephron atrophy, others suggest it is completely reversible [36, 37].

The effect of nontoxic amounts of lithium on glomerular filtration is generally much less than its effect on tubular function [28, 37–41]. When present, reduction of glomerular filtration rate is usually very slight.

Nephrotic syndrome is a rare adverse effect that can occur at therapeutic lithium levels [42]. In all reported cases, lithium discontinuation alone or combined with diuretics, hemodialysis, or prednisone resulted in improvement. In a 3-year prospective study of lithium-treated patients, a small but significant increase in urine protein excretion was found [43]. However, protein excretion remained within the normal range in all but a few and was not clinically meaningful.

Renal tubular acidosis (RTA), apparently related to lithium, has been described [44, 45]. Incomplete distal RTA induced by lithium is very slight and not of clinical importance. However, lithium-treated patients with other conditions or medications producing acidosis or those with urinary acidification defects may be at increased risk.

Little information exists regarding the use of lithium in patients with preexisting glomerulonephritis, pyelonephritis or tubulointerstitial disease. Whether those with preexisting kidney damage from other causes are more sensitive to lithium's nephrotoxic effects is not known, but it would be prudent to assume this to be the case.

While lithium is contraindicated in acute renal failure, it has been safely prescribed in patients with chronic renal failure [46]. When used in this setting, lithium should be prescribed in conservative doses with close monitoring of serum levels and renal function. We suggest maintaining serum lithium levels between 0.6 and 0.8 mEq/l. While lower serum lithium levels may be safer for kidney function, patients may be at higher risk for relapse of their mood disorder. Creatinine clearance should be evaluated before initiating lithium treatment and every 3–6 months thereafter. Whether such patients are at higher risk for further renal impairment caused by lithium is not known.

Lithium has been safely used in patients on hemodialysis [47–50] and continuous ambulatory peritoneal dialysis [51]. If other antimanic treatment options are not feasible and lithium is to be used in a patient on hemodialysis, we recommend that it be administered either in the dialysate or as a single oral dose following each dialysis. Administration of lithium in the dialysate may be preferable to oral dosing in those on peritoneal dialysis [51]. Initially, serum lithium levels should be monitored several times per week, and patients should be closely monitored for signs and symptoms of lithium intoxication.

Several reports describe the safe use of lithium after renal transplantation [52, 53]. However, acute tubular necrosis after cadaveric transplant presents a highly unstable situation with changing renal function resulting in wide fluctuations in lithium levels. Transplant patients are typically taking corticosteroids and/or cyclosporine for immunosuppression. Because methylprednisolone decreases fractional tubular reabsorption of lithium in rats [54] and cyclosporine has been shown to decrease fractional excretion of lithium [55, 56], lithium dosage adjustment may be necessary when using these drug combinations. In general, because of the renal effects of lithium described above, preferential consideration should be given to the use of carbamazepine and valproate for the treatment of manic patients with kidney disease.

Carbamazepine
Although albuminuria, glycosuria, increased blood urea nitrogen, microscopic deposits in urine, and acute renal failure have been reported with carbamazepine, significant effects on the kidney appear to be extremely rare [57].

Acute renal failure in a carbamazepine-treated patient was accompanied by granulomatous angiitis and severe eosinophilia, and was thought to be an idiosyncratic hypersensitivity reaction [58]. It is not known whether those with preexisting kidney disease are at higher risk for the development of carbamazepine-induced renal dysfunction.

Valproate

Valproate does not appear to affect renal structure or function. Valproate is extensively metabolized, but only 1–3% is renally excreted [59]. Although no data exist regarding the use of valproate in patients with preexisting kidney disease, valproate can probably be safely used in such patients with close monitoring of serum valproate levels and renal function.

Treatment of Mania in the Presence of Cardiovascular Disease

Lithium

T-wave flattening or inversion of no clinical consequence, the most comon electrocardiographic change associated with therapeutic lithium levels, has been reported in 13–100% of patients treated [60–63]. Sinus node dysfunction (marked sinus bradycardia, sinus arrest, sinoatrial block, and bradycardia/tachycardia), although uncommon, is the most frequently occurring lithium-related conduction defect, and may be secondary to the combination of lithium and a vulnerable conduction system [64, 65]. Few data exist linking lithium at therapeutic doses with other arrhythmias. Lithium toxicity may be associated with sinoatrial block, atrioventricular (AV) block, bradyarrhythmias, bundle branch block, ventricular tachycardia and ventricular-fibrillation [66]. The cautious use of lithium in the presence of preexisting cardiac arrhythmias appears reasonable given an appropriate psychiatric indication.

The association between lithium and myocarditis is tenuous, as is the relationship between lithium and sudden cardiac death. Because of a potentially increased risk of conduction disturbances and arrhythmias, some consider acute myocardial infarction a temporary contraindication to lithium use. Lithium has been safely used in a patient undergoing coronary artery bypass graft, but caution would certainly be indicated in such situations [67].

Thiazide diuretics induce increased distal tubular sodium loss, resulting in increased proximal tubular lithium absorption. Increased serum lithium levels and signs of intoxication have been described with combined lithium/thiazide use [68, 69]. The combined use of lithium and potassium-sparing diuretics has also been associated with increased serum lithium levels. Acetazolamide, a

carbamazepine treatment, have not been a problem. There is no evidence to suggest that those with preexisting skin disease or hair loss are at higher risk for development of valproate-related dermatologic effects.

Treatment of Mania in the Presence of Disorders of Carbohydrate Metabolism

Lithium
While several authors have reported lithium-induced decreases in glucose metabolism [96–99], others have reported apparent lithium-related hypoglycemia and increased glucose tolerance [100, 101]. Because lithium has been associated with increased, decreased, and unchanged glucose tolerance [102, 103], firm conclusions regarding lithium's effect on carbohydrate metabolism cannot be drawn. Patients with preexisting abnormalities of carbohydrate metabolism may be at increased risk for further abnormalities when treated with lithium and blood glucose should be more closely monitored.

Carbamazepine
There are no known effects of carbamazepine on carbohydrate metabolism nor evidence to suggest patients with preexisting disorders of carbohydrate metabolism are at risk for worsening when treated with carbamazepine.

Valproate
Hyperglycemia has been rarely reported in association with valproate treatment. Whether patients with preexisting disorders of carbohydrate metabolism are at higher risk for development of valproate-induced hyperglycemia is not known, but we would recommend such patients be more closely monitored.

Treatment of Mania in the Presence of Respiratory Disease

Lithium
In a study of 8 normal males, a significantly decreased response to mouth-occlusion pressure was found in subjects on lithium compared with controls [104]. We suggest that lithium be used cautiously in patients with chronic obstructive pulmonary disease (COPD). Several reports suggest lithium may have a beneficial effect in asthma [105, 106]. Although it is not clear whether it is truly beneficial to asthmatic patients, there is no evidence that lithium results in worsening.

In two studies with normal volunteers [107, 108], both aminophylline and theophylline were shown to significantly increase lithium excretion, particularly at higher theophylline levels. Concurrent use of lithium and theophylline may be associated with a decrease in serum lithium levels while theophylline discontinuation may result in increased levels and possible lithium toxicity.

Carbamazepine

Several cases of acute pulmonary hypersensitivity pneumonitis characterized by diffuse pulmonary infiltrates, skin rash and eosinophilia associated with carbamazepine treatment have been described [109–111a]. Because mycoplasma pneumonia titers were elevated in 1 patient and sputum culture was positive for mycobacterium tuberculosis in another, a causal link between carbamazepine and pneumonitis has not been definitively established. Some suggest the presence of preexisting pulmonary infection may increase the risk for development of drug-related acute pulmonary hypersensitivity pneumonitis. Carbamazepine treatment may result in decreased theophylline serum levels.

Valproate

There are no known effects of valproate on the lung. The use of valproate in patients with preexisting pulmonary disease appears reasonable given an appropriate psychiatric indication.

Treatment of Mania in the Presence of Gastrointestinal Disease

Lithium

Gastrointestinal side effects including anorexia, nausea, vomiting, loose stools, and abdominal pain are common early in lithium treatment. These effects may be minimized by taking fewer tablets or capsules at a time, taking medication with meals to slow absorption, or using sustained-release preparations. There is no evidence that lithium exacerbates preexisting ulcer disease.

Whether gastrointestinal disease alters lithium absorption has not been formally studies. Both vomiting and diarrhea could be expected to reduce absorption although associated dehydration might also increase the risk of lithium intoxication. The transfer of lithium in and out of the gastrointestinal tract is actually quite complex with lithium being returned to the gut through saliva, bile, pancreatic juice, and intestinal excretion. The net transfer, however, is in the direction of absorption and only a small portion of lithium is excreted in the feces. In the presence of acute gastrointestinal illness, temporary discontinuation of lithium is often indicated.

Carbamazepine

Early in treatment, carbamazepine may be associated with nausea and vomiting, diarrhea, stomatitis and glossitis. Generally, these side effects are mild and transient. Whether those with preexisting gastrointestinal disease are at higher risk for the development of carbamazepine-related gastrointestinal effects or worsening of preexisting gastrointestinal disease is not known. Such patients may benefit from gradual dosage increases and/or taking medication with meals to slow absorption.

Increased carbamazepine levels have been reported after the addition of cimetidine but not ranitidine. While others have found no change in carbamazepine levels after cimetidine addition, we recommend close monitoring for signs of carbamazepine toxicity when cimetidine is added to a stable carbamazepine regimen.

Valproate

Anorexia, nausea, and vomiting are common early side effects of valproic acid, but these effects are attenuated with the use of divalproex sodium (enteric-coated preparation). Pancreatitis and pancreatic pseudocyst are rare side effects of valproate. Whether patients with preexisting gastrointestinal or pancreatic disease are at greater risk for exacerbation when treated with valproate is not known, but we would advise consideration of an alternative antimanic agent in those with a history of pancreatic disorders.

Treatment of Mania in the Presence of Hepatic Disease

Lithium

Based on several early studies undertaken to investigate lithium's side effect profile, lithium has been assumed to have no hepatic side effects. However, lithium's effects on the liver have not been thoroughly investigated. Although lithium is not contraindicated in those with preexisting hepatic disease, its effects on hepatic function in such patients are unknown. We recommend liver function evaluation at baseline and at regular intervals in such patients, at least during the first few months of lithium treatment. In those with preexisting liver disease, lithium is likely to be safer than either carbamazepine or valproate (see below). In the presence of liver failure, lithium use would be complicated by the instability of the medical condition.

Carbamazepine

Mild increases in liver enzymes are common in patients treated with carbamazepine. Of greater concern is the idiosyncratic and unpredictable development of severe, potentially fatal, hepatotoxicity [111b]. In such cases, liver biopsy often reveals granulomatous hepatitis with cholangitis and cholestasis. Elderly patients may be more susceptible to severe carbamazepine-induced hepatotoxicity. Whether those with preexisting liver disease are also at higher risk is not known, but it would be prudent to assume this to be the case and to regularly monitor liver function tests in such patients.

Valproate

Mild, transient increases in hepatic enzymes, not usually accompanied by clinical symptoms of hepatic dysfunction, occur in up to 44% of valproate-treated patients. Fatal hepatotoxicity is rare, idiosyncratic and unrelated to dose. Children under age 2 on several antiepileptic drugs are at highest risk (1 in 500) for fatal hepatotoxicity. In addition, hepatic failure developed without any history of valproate treatment in siblings of at least 3 patients who died from valproate-related hepatotoxicity [112]. Because of decreased use in high-risk patients and increased use in lower-risk patients, the overall rate of severe valproate-related hepatotoxicity has decreased from 1 in 10,000 between 1978 and 1984 to 1 in 49,000 between 1985 and 1986 [112]. Rates are considerably lower when valproate is used as monotherapy. Some believe the mechanism for severe hepatotoxicity is aberrant cytochrome P-450-dependent valproate metabolism resulting in production of a toxic metabolite. It is recommended that clinicians avoid administering valproate to patients with preexisting liver disease or a family history of childhood hepatic disease. Because of similarities between valproate-related hepatotoxicity and Reye's syndrome, avoidance of concomitant salicylate use is also recommended.

Treatment of Mania in the Presence of Disorders of Calcium Metabolism

Lithium

Mild elevations of serum calcium and parathyroid hormone (PTH) without clinical manifestations have been observed in lithium-treated patients [113–116]. Several investigators have proposed that a higher serum calcium level is necessary in the presence of lithium for suppression of PTH secretion. Parathyroid adenomas, which may be coincidental or related to preexisting pathology, occur infrequently during lithium treatment. Whether patients with preexisting hyperparathyroidism are at increased risk during lithium treatment is not known. For such patients, we recommend regular evaluation of serum calcium.

Bone mineral content may be slightly reduced in lithium-treated patients, but this may be associated with the diagnosis of bipolar disorder rather than lithium treatment [117–119]. Whether children, adolescents, menopausal females, or patients with preexisting metabolic bone disease are at risk for lithium-induced bone changes has not been investigated. In the absence of compelling evidence for clinically significant effects on bone mineral content, we feel the use of lithium is safe in such patients. If children and young adolescents require lithium, we recommend that careful height and weight records be maintained, but we do not feel that monitoring of bone density by obtaining periodic hand radiographs is a necessary part of routine clinical practice.

Carbamazepine

Carbamazepine has been associated with decreased serum calcium, increased alkaline phosphatase, and decreased 25-OH vitamin D [120, 121a]. Symptomatic osteomalacia is rare, and has generally occurred in institutionalized epileptic patients taking large doses of carbamazepine and other anticonvulsants for many years. Whether patients with preexisting metabolic bone disease are at higher risk for carbamazepine-induced effects on calcium metabolism is not known. If children and adolescents are to be treated with carbamazepine, carefull height and weight records should be maintained.

Valproate

Valproate does not appear to affect calcium metabolism. The use of valproate in patients with preexisting disorders of calcium metabolism or metabolic bone disease appears reasonable.

Treatment of Mania in the Presence of Neurological Disease

Lithium

Lithium produces a variety of effects on the nervous system ranging from fatigue, muscle weakness, and fine hand tremor, to impaired consciousness, muscle fasciculations, coma, and death. In general, severe neurological effects occur at substantially elevated serum lithium levels, although neurotoxicity, especially in the elderly, has occasionally been described at therapeutic levels [121b, c]. Lithium has been safely used to treat behavioral changes in patients with structural brain damage as well as aggressive outbursts in elderly patients with dementia. Those with preexisting neurological disease are probably at higher risk for the development of neurological side effects when treated with lithium, but whether they are also at increased risk for severe neurotoxicity is not well established. Nonetheless, it would be prudent to assume this to be true. We would recommend such patients be maintained on lower serum lithium levels and carefully monitored for early signs of neurotoxicity.

Some, but not all, animal studies showed that lithium decreases seizure threshold. Reports of lithium use in epileptic patients are mixed with improvement, worsening, and no change in seizure activity described. Given the appropriate indication, we feel that the use of lithium in an epileptic patient whose seizures are well controlled with anticonvulsant medication is reasonable.

The symptoms of lithium intoxication are primarily neurological. When permanent neurological damage occurs, it is often cerebellar in nature (ataxia, dysarthria, intention tremor). While neurotoxicity has been described in some patients being treated with therapeutic amounts of lithium and carbamazepine, these drugs are usually well tolerated when combined.

Carbamazepine

Neurological phenomena comprise half of all carbamazepine side effect complaints [122] and include drowsiness, dizziness, diplopia, blurred vision, ataxia, and nystagmus. Usually, these side effects are transient and dose dependent. Elderly patients and those with underlying brain damage are at higher risk for development of carbamazepine-related neurological side effects. Neurotoxicity can be minimized by prescribing low initial doses with very gradual dosage increases and careful monitoring for neurological effects. Manic patients with underlying seizure disorders may benefit from the anticonvulsant effects of carbamazepine. However, there are a few reports of patients with generalized nonconvulsive seizures who developed convulsions when treated with carbamazepine.

Drug interactions may occur in patients with preexisting seizure disorders on other anticonvulsants. Through its enzyme-inducing properties, carbamazepine may accelerate the metabolism of phenytoin, phenobarbital, primidone, and valproate. Conversely, hepatic metabolism of carbamazepine may be increased by phenytoin, phenobarbital, and primidone.

Valproate

Sedation may occur early in valproate treatment and is often dose-related. Mild tremor resembling benign essential tremor occurs in 2–3% of treated patients and is often dose-related [81]. Stupor may rarely occur, but is likely the result of drug interactions between valproate and other antiepileptic drugs. Incoordination and ataxia, when they occur, are usually the result of multidrug therapy. Manic patients with an underlying seizure disorder may benefit from the anticonvulsant effects of valproate.

Two patients with multiple sclerosis were treated with valproate for 'organic brain syndrome' [123]. Both benefited from valproate administration, and neither experienced increased confusion during treatment.

Serum levels of phenobarbital and primidone are increased in many patients during concurrent valproate treatment. Valproate lowers phenytoin blood levels but increases free drug levels by displacing phenytoin from protein binding sites. Serum levels of carbamazepine and of its epoxide metabolite are increased during concurrent valproate treatment. Because of liver enzyme induction, higher valproate doses may be required to obtain therapeutic serum concentrations during concurrent treatment with phenobarbital, phenytoin, primidone, or carbamazepine.

Treatment of Mania in the Presence of Hematologic Disease

Lithium

The most consistent hematological effect induced by lithium is benign, reversible granulocytosis representing a true proliferative response rather than demargination of cells into the circulation. This adverse effect has been turned to advantage in the treatment of leukopenic conditions such as Felty's syndrome and neutropenia induced by myelosuppressive cancer chemotherapy. While there have been some reports of increased platelet count and increased platelet aggregation in lithium-treated patients, these effects have not been shown to be of clinical importance. In addition, lithium has no clinically important effects on red blood cell counts or coagulation. Whether those with preexisting hematological disease are at higher risk for the development of adverse effects on lithium is not known.

Carbamazepine

Benign transient leukopenia occurs in approximately 10% of carbamazepine-treated patients and is persistent in approximately 2% [81]. More severe hematologic effects, aplastic anemia and agranulocytosis, are rare, idiosyncratic, and unpredictable. Development of lymphoproliferative disorders has been rarely reported in carbamazepine-treated patients. Whether those with preexisting hematologic disease are at higher risk for the development of benign or severe hematologic effects on carbamazepine is not known, but regular monitoring of blood counts is recommended in such patients. If the total white blood count falls below 2,500–3,000/µl or the absolute neutrophil count falls below 1,500/µl, carbamazepine discontinuation should be considered.

Valproate

Thrombocytopenia and impairment of platelet function may occur during valproate treatment. Leukopenia ($< 4,000/mm^3$) occurs in approximately 3–8% [80]. While statistically significant, these changes are generally without clinical consequence. Severe hematologic toxicity develops very rarely, is idiosyncratic and unpredictable, and occurs less frequently than with carbamazepine treatment. Age may be a risk factor for the development of aplastic anemia on valproate.

Treatment of Mania in the Presence of Cancer

Lithium

Lithium attenuates chemotherapy-induced granulocytopenia regardless of the chemotherapeutic agent or the site of cancer. Some have reported decreased infections, infection-related deaths [124], and number of readmissions for febrile complications [125, 126], presumably a benefit from lithium treatment. Despite concern that myelogenous leukemic cells sensitive to colony-stimulating factor may proliferate when leukemic patients are treated with lithium, epidemiologic studies suggest lithium does not increase the risk of leukemia [127–129]. There is no evidence that lithium treatment results in exacerbation or recurrence of other types of cancer. Because of its favorable hematologic profile when compared with carbamazepine and valproate, lithium should receive preferential consideration for the treatment of mania in those taking myelosuppressive chemotherapeutic agents.

Carbamazepine

While there are no data suggesting carbamazepine treatment worsens or increases the recurrence risk for any form of cancer, the hematologic side effects of carbamazepine (see above) are of concern in patients on myelosuppressive chemotherapeutic agents. If alternative antimanic treatments have been exhausted, carbamazepine should be used cautiously with frequent, regular evaluation of blood counts.

Carbamazepine intoxication and increased carbamazepine serum levels have occurred when propoxyphene (Darvon) was added to a stable carbamazepine regimen. Cancer patients taking propoxyphene for pain may be at risk for development of carbamazepine toxicity.

Valproate

Hematologic side effects of valproate (see above) and myelosuppressive effects of chemotherapy may be additive. Unless alternative antimanic treatments have been exhausted, valproate should not be considered for manic patients taking myelosuppressive chemotherapeutic agents. There is no evidence suggesting that valproate worsens or increases the risk of recurrence for any form of cancer.

Treatment of Mania in the Presence of Infectious Disease

Lithium
Lithium has been shown to inhibit viral replication and to stimulate protective host immune responses to viruses. Several studies have suggested that lithium may be effective in the treatment of herpes simplex infections [130–132]. Although it is not known whether lithium possesses anti-human immunodeficiency virus (HIV) effects, lithium may be beneficial in the treatment of zidovudine-induced neutropenia. In addition, lithium may be beneficial in the treatment of secondary mania induced by zidovudine treatment, opportunistic infections, or central nervous system HIV infection [133]. In a recent study of lithium's antiviral and immunologic effects in HIV-infected patients, 8 of 10 developed symptoms of lithium toxicity at serum levels between 0.5 and 1.5 mEq/l. We recommend that HIV-infected patients treated with lithium be maintained at lower serum lithium levels and closely monitored for toxicity [134].

While an earlier report [135] described elevated lithium levels and toxic symptoms in a patient who had started tetracycline treatment 2 days before, a study of 14 healthy volunteers [136] revealed slightly, but significantly lower serum lithium levels on lithium/tetracycline treatment than on lithium alone. The drug combination appears unlikely to result in significant problems. Most nonsteroidal antiinflammatory agents (with the exception of aspirin and sulindac) reduce renal lithium clearance and may increase serum lithium levels. There have been 3 cases reported in which metronidazole (Flagyl) treatment was associated with a total increase in serum lithium level and reduced renal function [137].

Carbamazepine
Carbamazepine may reduce serum concentrations of IgA and IgM [81]. However, there is no evidence to suggest that carbamazepine-treated patients whose blood counts are within the normal range are at increased risk for infection.

The hepatic metabolism of carbamazepine may be inhibited by two macrolide antibiotics, erythromycin and triacetyloleandomycin with resultant toxicity. Carbamazepine toxicity has also developed when isoniazid was added to a stable carbamazepine regimen [84].

Valproate
While some have described IgA deficiency in some valproate-treated patients, others have found no changes in immunoglobulin levels. However, there are no data to suggest that valproate-treated patients whose blood counts are within the normal range are at increased risk for infection.

Treatment of Mania in Surgical Patients

Lithium

When lithium-treated patients require surgery, involved physicians must be aware of the potential for dehydration and resulting lithium intoxication, drug interactions between lithium and anesthetic agents, and recurrence of mania or depression. Ideally, lithium should be discontinued several days before the procedure. Because patients with lithium-induced polyuria and polydipsia may become rapidly dehydrated when fluid-restricted, parenteral fluids may be necessary the night before surgery [138]. Since lithium-induced polyuria may persist despite drug discontinuation, careful attention to parenteral fluid replacement will be necessary to prevent dehydration.

Interactions between lithium and inhalational anesthetics are very rare. Lithium may prolong the action of depolarizing (e.g. succinylcholine) and nondepolarizing (e.g. pancuronium) neuromuscular blocking agents, resulting in prolonged anesthesia [139]. A nerve stimulator may be helpful for titration of muscle relaxant dosage. Lithium may increase the duration of activity of barbiturates and benzodiazepines [140]. Nonsteroidal antiinflammatory agents used for postoperative analgesia reduce renal clearance of lithium, resulting in elevation of serum lithium levels [139].

In order to prevent recurrence of mania, lithium treatment should be resumed as soon as oral intake is resumed and kidney function, electrolyte balance and hydration status have normalized. Occasionally, the preoperative dosage will be less well tolerated during convalescence so that dosage reduction may be necessary.

Carbamazepine

A 16-year-old patient taking carbamazepine for a partial complex seizure disorder underwent cardiothoracic surgery for Wolff-Parkinson-White syndrome [141]. He suffered an intraoperative myocardial infarction and developed pulmonary edema and carbamazepine toxicity postoperatively. Serum carbamazepine level was 18.9 μg/ml. The authors suggest carbamazepine toxicity may have resulted from changes in protein binding and altered hepatic function.

Few additional data are available regarding carbamazepine-treated patients who undergo surgery. We recommend carbamazepine discontinuation several days before surgery and resumption as soon as safely possible postoperatively, provided liver function is normal. As described earlier, carbamazepine may accelerate barbiturate metabolism. If used for postoperative analgesia, propoxyphene may increase carbamazepine levels. Due to hepatic enzyme induction, carbamazepine may increase metabolism of warfarin anticoagulants.

Valproate

A 12-year-old patient with cerebral palsy taking valproate, phenytoin, and phenobarbital for a seizure disorder developed excessive intraoperative bleeding during a procedure for adductor tendon hip release [142]. Hematocrit, platelet count, PT, and PTT were normal preoperatively. The authors suggest that intraoperative bleeding was a result of valproate-induced impairment of platelet function and recommend preoperative determination of bleeding time in such patients.

There is little additional information available regarding valproate-treated patients undergoing surgery. We recommend valproate discontinuation several days before surgery and resumption of treatment as soon as safely possible. Platelet function must be thoroughly evaluated preoperatively, and physicians should be aware of the possibility that postoperative bleeding may increase following resumption of valproate treatment. As described above, serum barbiturate levels may be elevated in valproate-treated patients.

Conclusion

Although lithium, carbamazepine, and valproate may be used safely to treat mania in the presence of most nonpsychiatric medical illnesses, close collaboration among all involved physicians is essential. Because there are few studies addressing the use of these medications in patients with concurrent medical illnesses, monitoring recommendations remain tentative. Further research in this area will allow recommendations to be based more on data than speculation.

References

1   Chou JCY: Recent advances in treatment of acute mania. J Clin Psychopharmacol 1991; 11:3–21.
2   Small JG: Anticonvulsants in affective disorders. Psychopharmacol Bull 1990;26:25–36.
3a Pope HG, McElroy SL, Keck PE, Hudson JI: Valproate in the treatment of acute mania. Arch Gen Psychiatry 1991;48:62–68.
3b Bowden CL, Brugger A, Percy J, Swann AG: Efficacy of valproate in acute mania. Continuing Medical Education Syllabus and Scientific Proceedings, American Psychiatric Association, 1993.
4   Schou M, Amdisen A, Jensen SE, Olsen T: Occurrence of goiter during lithium treatment. Br Med J 1968;iii:710–713.
5   Emerson C, Dyson W, Utiger R: Serum thyrotropin and thyroxine concentrations in patients receiving lithium carbonate. J Clin Endocrinol Metab 1973;36:338–346.
6   Baldessarini R, Lipinski J: Lithium salts: 1970–1975. Ann Intern Med 1975;83:527–533.

7   Piziak V, Sellman J, Othmer E: Lithium and hypothyroidism. J Clin Psychiatry 1978; 39: 709–711.

8   Sedvall G, Jonsson B, Peterson V: Evidence of an altered thyroid function in man during treatment with lithium carbonate. Acta Psychiatr Scand 1969;207(supp):59–67.

9   Cooper T, Simpson G: Preliminary report of a longitudinal study in the effects of lithium on iodine metabolism. Curr Ter Res 1969;11:603–608.

10   Myers D, Carter R, Burns B, Armond A, Hussain SB, Chengapa VK: A prospective study of the effects of lithium on thyroid function and on the prevalence of antithyroid antibodies. Psychol Med 1985;15:55–61.

11   Fieve R, Platman S: Lithium and thyroid function in manic-depressive psychosis. Am J Psychiatry 1968;125:119–122.

12   Lazarus JH, John R, Bennie EH, Chalmers RJ, Crockett G: Lithium therapy and thyroid function. A long-term study. Psychol Med 1981;11:85–92.

13   Martino E, Placid G, Sardano G, Mariotti S, Fornaro P, Pinchera A, Baschieri: High incidence of goiter in patients treated with lithium carbonate. Ann Endocrinol 1982;43:269–276.

14   Yassa R, Saunders A, Nastase C: Lithium-induced thyroid disorders: A prevalence study. J Clin Psychiatry 1988;49:14–16.

15   Calabrese JR, Gulledge AD, Hahn K, Skwerer R, Kotz M, Schumacher OP, Gupta MK, Krupp N, Gold PW: Autoimmune thyroiditis in manic-depressive patients treated with lithium. Am J Psychiatry 1985;142:1318–1321.

16   Smigan L, Wahlin A, Jacobsson L, Von Knorring L: Lithium therapy and thyroid function tests: A prospective study. Neuropsychobiology 1984;11:39–43.

17a   Maarbjerg K, Vestergaard P, Schou M: Changes in serum thyroxine (T4) and serum thyroid stimulating hormone (TSH) during prolonged lithium treatment. Acta Psychiatr Scand 1987; 75:217–221.

17b   Bocchetta A, Bernandi F, Burnai C, Pedditzi M, Loviselli A, Velluzzi F, Martino E, Del Zompo M: The cause of thyroid abnormalities during lithium treatment: A two-year follow-up study. Acta Psychiatr Scand 1992;86:38–41.

18   Amdisen A, Andersen CJ: Lithium treatment and thyroid function: A survey of 237 patients in long-term lithium treatment. Pharmacopsychiatry 1982;15:149–155.

19   Schoenberg M, Ts'o TOT, Meisel AN: Graves' disease manifesting after maintenance lithium. J Nerv Ment Dis 1979;167:575–577.

20   Rosser R: Thyrotoxicosis and lithium. Br J Psychiatry 1976;128:61–66.

21   Hartzband PI, Solomon DH: Hyperthyroidism: Choosing the appropriate therapy. Drug Ther Rev 1983;13:27–42.

22   Hedley J, Turner JG, Brownlie BE, Sadler WA: Low dose lithium-carbamizole in the treatment of thyrotoxicosis. Aust N Z J Med 1978;8:628–630.

23   Turner JB, Brownlie BEW, Sadler WA, Jensen CH: An evaluation of lithium as an adjunct to carbamizole treatment in acute thyrotoxicosis. Acta Endocrinol (Copenh) 1976;83:86–92.

24   Turner JG, Brownlie BEW, Rogers TGH: Lithium as an adjunct to radioiodine therapy for thyrotoxicosis. Lancet 1976;i:614–615.

25a   Kramlinger KG, Post RM: The addition of lithium carbonate to carbamazepine: Hematological and thyroid effects. Am J Psychiatry 1990;147:615–620.

25b   Herman R, Abarranek E, Mikalanskas KM, Post RM, Jimerson DC: The effects of carbamazepine on resting metabolic rate of thyroid function in depressed patients. Biol Psychiatry 1991;29:779–788.

26   Hegedus L, Hansen JM, Luhdorf K, Perrild H, Feldt-Rasmussen U, Kampmann JP: Increased frequency of goitre in epileptic patients on long-term phenytoin or carbamazepine treatment. Clin Endocrinol 1985;23:423–429.

27   Fichsel H, Knopfle G: Effects of anticonvulsant drugs on thyroid hormones in epileptic children. Epilepsia 1978;19:323–336.

28   Bendz H: Kidney function in lithium-treated patients: A literature survey. Acta Psychiatr Scand 1983;68:303–324.

29   Gelenberg AJ, Kane JM, Keller MB, Lavori PW, Rosenbaum JF, Cole K, Lavelle J: Compari-

son of standard and low serum levels of lithium for maintenance treatment of bipolar disorder. N Engl J Med 1989;321:1489–1493.

30 Simon NM, Garber E, Arieff A: Persistent nephrogenic diabetes insipidus after lithium carbonate. Ann Intern Med 1977;86:446–447.

31 Bucht G, Wahlin A: Renal concentrating capacity in long-term lithium treatment after withdrawal of lithium. Acta Med Scand 1980;207:309–314.

32 Rabin EZ, Garston RG, Weir RV, Posen GA: Persistent nephrogenic diabetes insipidus associated with long-term lithium carbonate treatment. Can Med Assoc J 1979;121:194–198.

33 Hansen HE, Hestbech J, Sorenson JL, Norgaard K, Heilskov J, Amdisen A: Chronic interstitial nephropathy in patients on long-term lithium treatment. Q J Med 1979;48:577–591.

34 Walker RG, Dowlin JP, Alcorn D, Ryan GB, Kincaid-Smith P: Renal pathology associated with lithium therapy. Pathology 1983;15:403–411.

35a Walker RG, Davies BM, Holwill BJ, Dowling JP, Kincaid-Smith P: A clinicopathological study of lithium nephrotoxicity. J Chron Dis 1982;35:685–695.

35b Walker RG: Lithium nephrotoxicity. Kidney Int 1993;44(suppl 42):93–98.

36 Burrows GD, Davies B, Kincaid-Smith P: Unique tubular lesion after lithium. Lancet 1978;i:1310.

37 Schou M: Effects of long-term lithium treatment on kidney function: An overview. J Psychiatr Res 1988;22:287–296.

38 Boton R, Gaviria M, Batlle DC: Prevalence, pathogenesis, and treatment of renal dysfunction associated with chronic lithium therapy. Am J Kidney Dis 1987;10:329–345.

39 Grof P, MacCrimmon DJ, Smith EKM, Daigle L, Saxena B, Varmar Grof E, Keitner G, Kenny J: Long-term lithium treatment and the kidney: Interim report on fifty patients. Can J Psychiatry 1980;25:535–544.

40 Vaamonde CA, Milian NE, Magrinat GS: Longitudinal evaluation of glomerular filtration rate during long-term lithium therapy. Am J Kidney Dis 1986;7:213–216.

41 Schou M, Vestergaard P: Prospective studies in a lithium cohort. 2. Renal function, water and electrolyte metabolism. Acta Psychiatr Scand 1988;78:427–443.

42 Wood IK, Parmelee DX, Foreman JW: lithium-induced nephrotic syndrome. Am J Psychiatry 1989;146:84–87.

43 Amsterdam JD, Jorkasky D, Potter L, Cox M: A prospective study of lithium-induced nephropathy: Preliminary results. Psychopharmacol Bull 1985;21:81–84.

44 Perez GO, Oster JR, Vaamonde CA: Incomplete syndrome of renal tubular acidosis induced by lithium carbonate. J Lab Clin Med 1975;86:386–394.

45 Ostrow DG, Coe FL, Wolpert EA: A study of renal function in patients treated with a flexible dose lithium regimen. J Psychiatr Treat Eval 1982;4:269–278.

46 Csernansky JG, Hollister LE: Using lithium in patients with cardiac and renal disease. Hosp Formul 1985;20:726–735.

47 Lippman SB, Manshadi MS, Gultekin A: Lithium in a patient with renal failure on hemodialysis. J Clin Psychiatry 1984;45:444.

48 Port FK, Kroll PD, Rosenzweig J: Lithium therapy during maintenance hemodialysis. Psychosomatics 1979;20:130–131.

49 Procci WR: Mania during maintenance hemodialysis successfully treated with oral lithium carbonate. J Nerv Ment Dis 1977;164:355–358.

50 Zetin M, Plon L, Vaziri N, Cramer M, Greco D: Lithium carbonate dose and serum level relationships in chronic hemodialysis patients. Am J Psychiatry 1981;138:1387–1388.

51 Flynn CT, Chandran PKG, Taylor MJ, Shadur CA: Intraperitoneal lithium administration for bipolar affective disorder in a patient on continuous ambulatory peritoneal dialysis. Int J Artif Organs 1987;10:105–107.

52 Koecheler JA, Canafax DM, Simmons RL, Najarian JS: Lithium dosing in renal allograft recipients with changing renal function. Drug Intell Clin Pharm 1986;20:623–624.

53 Blazer DG, Petrie WM, Wilson WP: Affective psychoses following renal transplant. Dis Nerv Syst 1976;37:663–667.

54 Imbs J-L, Singer L, Danion J-M: Effects of indomethacin and methylprednisolone on renal elimination of lithium in the rat. Int Pharmacopsychiatry 1980;5:143–149.

55   Vincent HH, Weimar W, Schalekamp MADH: Effect of cyclosporine in fractional excretion of lithium and potassium in kidney transplant recipients. Kidney Int 1987;31:1048.

56   Dieperink H, Leyssac PP, Kemp E, Starklint H, Frandsen NE, Tuede N, Moller J, Buchler Fredericksen P, Rossing N: Nephrotoxicity of cyclosporin A in humans: Effects on glomerular filtration and tubular reabsorption rates. Eur J Clin Invest 1947;17:493–496.

57   Physicians' Desk Reference: PDR, ed 45. Oradell, Medical Economics Company, 1991.

58   Imai H, Nakamoto Y, Kirokawa M, Akihama T, Miura AB: Carbamazepine-induced granulomatous necrotizing angiitis with acute renal failure. Nephron 1989;51:405–408.

59   Kandrotas RJ, Love JM, Gal P, Oles KS: The effect of hemodialysis and hemoperfusion on serum valproic acid concentration. Neurology 1990;40:1456–1458.

60   Jefferson JW, Greist JH: The cardiovascular effects and toxicity of lithium; in Davis JM, Greenblatt D (eds): Psychopharmacology Update: New and Neglected Areas. New York, Grune & Stratton, 1979, pp 65–79.

61   Mitchell JE, Mackenzie TB: Cardiac effects of lithium therapy in man: A review. J Clin Psychiatry 1982;43:47–51.

62   Risch SC, Groom GP, Janowsky DS: The effects of psychotropic drugs on the cardiovascular system. J Clin Psychiatry 1982;43:16–31.

63   Bucht G, Smigan L, Wahlin A, Eriksson P: ECG changes during lithium therapy: A prospective study. Acta Med Scand 1984;216:101–104.

64   Brady HR, Horgan JH: Lithium and the heart: Unanswered questions. Chest 1988;93:166–169.

65   Hagman A, Arnman K, Ryden L: Syncope caused by lithium treatment: Report on two cases and a prospective investigation of lithium-induced sinus node dysfunction. Acta Med Scand 1979;205:467–471.

66   Marin CA, Dickson LR, Kuo C: Heart and blood vessels; in Johnson FN (ed): Depression and Mania: Modern Lithium Therapy, Oxford/Washington, IRL Press, 1987, pp 213–218.

67   Wolpert EA, Margul B, Replogle R, et al: Coronary artery bypass in a patient on lithium carbonate prophylaxis. J Nerv Ment Dis 1982;170:181–184

68   Jefferson JW, Kalin NH: Serum lithium levels and long-term diuretic use. JAMA 1979;241:1134–1136.

69   Himmelhoch JM, Poust RI, Mallinger AG, Hanin I, Neil JF: Adjustment of lithium dose during lithium-chlorothiazide therapy. Clin Pharmacol Ther 1977;22:225–227.

70   Saffer D, Coppen A: Frusemide: A safe diuretic during lithium therapy? J Affective Disord 1983;5:289–292.

71   Price WA, Giannini AJ: Neurotoxicity caused by lithium-verapamil synergism. J Clin Pharmacol 1986;26:717–719.

72   Price WA, Shalley JE: Lithium-verapamil toxicity in the elderly. J Am Geriatr Soc 1987;35:177–178.

73   Cooper SJ, Kelly JG, Johnston GD, Copeland S, King DJ, McDevitt DG: Pharmacodynamics and pharmacokinetic of digoxin in the presence of lithium. Br J Clin Pharmacol 1984;18:21–25.

74   Byrd GJ: Methyldopa and lithium carbonate: Suspected interaction. JAMA 1975;233:320.

75   O'Regan JB: Adverse interaction of lithium carbonate and methyldopa. Can Med Assoc J 1976;115:385–386.

76   Osanloo E, Deglin JH: Interaction of lithium and methyldopa. Ann Intern Med 1980; 92:433–434.

77   Yassa R: Lithium-methyldopa interaction. Can Med Assoc J 1986;134:141–142.

78   Walker N, White K, Tornatore F, Boyd JL, Cohen JL: Lithium-methyldopa interactions in normal subjects. Drug Intell Clin Pharm 1980;14:638–639.

79   Douste-Blazy P, Rostin M, Livarek B, et al: Angiotensin converting enzyme inhibitors and lithium treatment. Lancet 1986;i:1448.

80a Gelenberg AJ: ACE inhibitors and lithium toxicity. Biol Ther Pschiatry 1988;11:43.

80b DasGupta K, Jefferson JW, Kobak KA, Greist JH: The effects of enalapril on serum lithium levels in healthy men. J Clin Psychiatry 1992;53:398–400.

81   Keranen T, Sivenius J: Side effects of carbamazepine, valproate, and clonazepam during long-term treatment of epilepsy. Acta Neurol Scand 1983;68(suppl 97):69–80.

82a Boesen F, Andersen EB, Jensen EK: Cardiac conduction disturbances during carbamazepine therapy. Acta Neurol Scand 1983;8:49–52.

82b Kasarskis EJ, Kuo C-S, Berger R, Nelson KR: Carbamazepine-induced cardiac dysfunction. Arch Intern Med 1992;152:186–191.

83a Terrence CF, Fromm G: Congestive heart failure during carbamazepine therapy. Ann Neurol 1980;8:200–201.

83b Kennebäck G, Bergfeldt L, Vallin H, Tomson T, Edhag O: Electrophysiologic effects and clinical hazards of carbamazepine treatment for neurologic disorders in patients with abnormalities of the cardiac conduction system. Am Heart J 1991;121:1421–1429.

84 Ciraulo DA, Slattery M, Shader RI: An overview of drug interactions of anticonvulsants commonly used in psychiatry, in: Ciraulo DA, Shader RI, Greenblatt DH, Creelman W (eds): Drug Interactions in Psychiatry. Baltimore, Williams & Wilkins, 1989, pp 181–233.

85 Remmer HI, Falk WE: Successful treatment of lithium-induced acne. J Clin Psychiatry 1986;47:48.

86 Lambert D, Dalac S: Skin, hair, and nails; in Johnson FN (ed): Depression and Mania: Modern Lithium Therapy. Oxford, IRL Press, 1987, pp 232–234.

87 Carter TN: The relationship of lithium carbonate to psoriasis. Psychosomatics 1972;13:325–327.

88 Skoven I, Thormann J: Lithium compound treatment and psoriasis. Arch Dermatol 1979;115:1185–1187.

89 Deandrea D, Walker N, Mehlmauer M, White K: Dermatological reactions to lithium: A critical review of the literature. J Clin Psychopharmacol 1982;2:199–204.

90 Callaway CL, Hendrie HC, Luby ED: Cutaneous conditions observed in patients during treatment with lithium. Am J Psychiatry 1968;124:1124–1125.

91 Jefferson JW, Greist JH, Diamond RL, Marcetich JR: Lithium and hair loss. Int DrugTher Newslett 1979;14:23.

92 Mortimer PS, Dawber RPR: Hair loss and lithium. Int J Dermatol 1984;23:603–604.

93 Boyle J, Burton JL, Faergemann J: Use of topical lithium succinate for seborrhoeic dermatitis. Br Med J 1986;292:28.

94 Fawcett RG: Erythema multiforme major in a patient treated with carbamazepine. J Clin Psychiatry 1987;48:416–417.

95 Chadwick D, Shaw MDM, Foy P Rawlins MD, Turnbull DM: Serum anticonvulsant concentrations and the risk of drug induced skin eruptions. J Neurol Neurosurg Psychiatry 1984;47:642–644.

96 Shopsin B, Stern S, Gershon S: Altered carbohydrate metabolism during treatment with lithium carbonate: Absence of diagnostic specificity in hospitalized psychiatric patients. Arch Gen Psychiatry 1972;26:566–571.

97 Muller-Oerlinghausen B, Passoth P-M, Poser W, Pudel V: Impaired glucose tolerance in long-term lithium-treated patients. Int Pharmacopsychiatry 1979;14:350–362.

98 Waziri R, Nelson J: Lithium in diabetes mellitus: A paradoxical response. J Clin Psychiatry 1978;39:623–625.

99 Kondziela JR, Kaufmann MW, Klein MJ: Diabetic ketoacidosis associated with lithium: Case report. J Clin Psychiatry 1985;46:492–493.

100 Vendsborg PB, Rafaelsen OJ: Lithium in man: Effect on glucose tolerance and serum electrolytes. Acta Psychiatr Scand 1973;49:601–610.

101 Vendsborg PB: Lithium and glucose tolerance in manic-melancholic patients. Acta Psychiatr Scand 1979;59:306–316.

102 Agbayewa MO: Glycosylated hemoglobin (risk of diabetes mellitus) in lithium therapy. Psychiatr J Univ Ottawa 1986;11:153–155.

103 Vestergaard P, Shou M: Does long-term lithium treatment induce diabetes mellitus? Neuropsychobiology 1987;17:130–132.

104 Weiner M, Chausow A, Wolpert E, Addingto W, Szidon P: Effects of lithium on the responses to added respiratory resistances. N Engl J Med 1983;308:319–322.

105 Nasr SJ, Atkins RW: Coincidental improvement in asthma during lithium treatment. Am J Psychiatry 1977;134:1042–1043.

106 Winig HR: More on lithium and asthma. Am J Psychiatry 1978;135:998.

107 Thomsen K, Schou M: Renal lithium excretion in man. Am J Physiol 1968;215:823–827.

108 Perry PJ, Calloway RA, Cook BL, Smith RE: Theophylline precipitated alterations of lithium clearance. Acta Psychiatr Scand 1984;69:528–537.

109 Stephan WC, Parks RD, Tempest B: Acute hypersensitivity pneumonitis associated with carbamazepine therapy. Chest 1978;74:463–464.

110 Cullinan SA, Bower GC: Acute pulmonary hypersensitivity to carbamazepine. Chest 1975;68: 580–581.

111a Barreiro B, Manresa F, Valldeperas J: Carbamazepine and the lung. Eur Respir J 1990;3: 930–931.

111b Forbes GM, Jeffrey GP, Shilkin KB, Reed WD: Carbamazepine hepatotoxicity: Another cause of the vanishing bile duct syndrome. Gastroenterology 1992;142:1385–1388.

112 Dreifuss FE, Langer DH, Moline KA, Maxwell JE: Valproic acid hepatic fatalities. II. US experience since 1984. Neurology 1989;39:201–207.

113 Christiansen C, Baastrup PC, Transbol I: Development of 'primary' hyperparathyroidism during lithium therapy: Longitudinal study. Neuropsychobiology 1980;6:280–283.

114 Labib MH: Lithium, hypercalcemia and hyperparathyroidism. Ann Clin Biochem 1987;24: 147–148.

115 McIntosh WB, Horn EH, Mathieson LM, Sumner D: The prevalence, mechanism and clinical significance of lithium-induced hypercalcaemia. Med Lab Sci 1987;44:115–118.

116 Franks RD, Dubovsky SL, Lifshitz ML, Coen P, Subryan V, Walker SH: Long-term lithium carbonate therapy causes hyperparathyroidism. Arch Gen Psychiatry 1982;39:1074–1077.

117 Christiansen C, Baastrup PC, Transbol I: Osteopenia and dysregulation of divalent cations in lithium-treated patients. Neuropsychobiology 1975;1:334–354.

118 Plenge P, Rafaelsen OF: Lithium effects on calcium, magnesium and phosphate in man: Effects on balance, bone mineral content, faecal and urinary excretion. Acta Psychiatr Scand 1982; 66:361–373.

119 Birch NJ: Bone side effects of lithium; in Johnson FN (ed): Handbook of Lithium Therapy. Lancaster, MTP Press, 1990, pp 365–371.

120 Tjellesen L, Christiansen C: Serum vitamin D metabolites in epileptic patients treated with 2 different anticonvulsants. Preliminary report. Acta Neurol Scand 1982;66:335–341.

121a O'Hare JA, Duggan B, O'Driscoll D, Callaghan N: Biochemical evidence for osteomalacia with carbamazepine therapy. Acta Neurol Scand 1980;62:282–286.

121b Foster JR: Use of lithium in elderly psychiatric patients: A review of the literature. Lithium 1992;3:77–93.

121c Bell AJ, Cole A, Eccleston D, Ferrier IN: Lithium neurotoxicity at normal therapeutic levels. Br J Psychiatry 1993;162:689–692.

122 Jefferson JW, Greist JH: Lithium carbonate and carbamazepine side effects; in Hales RE, Frances AJ (eds): American Psychiatric Association Annual Review. Washington, American Psychiatric Press, 1987, vol 6, pp 746–780.

123 Kahn D, Stevenson E, Douglas CJ: Effect of sodium valproate in three patients with organic brain syndromes. Am J Psychiatry 1988;145:1010–1011.

124 Lyman GH, Williams CC, Preston D: The use of lithium carbonate to reduce infection and leukopenia during systemic chemotherapy. N Engl J Med 1980;302:257–260.

125 Turner AR, MacDonald RN, McPherson TA: Reduction of chemotherapy-induced neutropenic complications with a short course of lithium carbonate. Clin Invest Med 1979;2:51–53.

126 Torti FM, Molin EM, Hannigan JF, Freiha FS: Lithium carbonate reduces episodes of neutropenic infection in patients receiving chemotherapy for testicular cancer. Clin Res 1984;32:423a.

127 Lyskowski J, Nasrallah HA: Lithium therapy and the risk for leukemia. Br J Psychiatry 1981;139:256.

128 Norton B, Whalley LJ: Mortality of a lithium-treated population. Br J Psychiatry 1984;145: 277–282.

129 Frenkel EP, Herbert V: Frequency of granulocytopenic leukemia in populations drinking highvs. low-lithium water. Clin Res 1974;22:390a.

130 Skinner GRB, Hartley C, Buchan A, Harper L, Gallimore P: The effects of lithium chloride on the replication of herpes simplex virus. Med Microbiol Immunol 1980, 168:139–148.

131 Patou G, Crow TJ, Taylor GR: The effects of psychotropic drugs on synthesis of DNA and the infectivity of herpes simplex virus. Biol Psychiatry 1986;21:1221–1225.

132 Amsterdam JD, Maislin G, Potter L, Giuntoli R, Koprowski H. Suppression of recurrent genital herpes infections with lithium carbonate: A randomized, placebo-controlled trial. Lithium 1991;2:17–25.

133 Schaerf FW: The use of lithium in HIV-1 infection. Int Drug Ther Newslett 1989;24:17–19.

134 Parenti DM, Simon GL, Scheib RG, Meyer WA, Sztein MB, Paxton H, DiGioia RA, Schulof RS: Effect of lithium carbonate in HIV-infected patients with immune dysfunction. J Acquir Immune Defic Syndr 1988;1:119–124.

135 McGennis AJ: Lithium carbonate and tetracycline interaction (letter). Br Med J 1978;i:1183.

136 Fankhauser MP, Lindon JL, Connolly B, Healey WJ: Evaluation of lithium-tetracycline interaction. Clin Pharm 1988;7:314–317.

137 Ayd FJ: Lithium and metronidazole interaction resulting in possible nephrotoxicity. Int Drug Ther Newslett 1987;22:33–34.

138 Schou M, Hippus H: Guidelines for patients receiving lithium treatment who require major surgery (letter). Br J Anaesth 1987;59:809–810.

139 Creelman W, Ciraulo DA, Shader RI: Lithium drug interactions; in Ciraulo DA, Shader RI, Greenblatt DJ, Creelman W (eds): Drug Interactions in Psychiatry. Baltimore, Willimas & Wilkins, 1989, pp 127–157.

140 Pottecher T, Ludes B, Lichnewsky M, Calon B: Surgery under lithium; in Johnson FN (ed): Depression and Mania: Modern Lithium Therapy. Oxford, IRL Press, 1987, pp 150–151.

141 Wright PS, Seifert CF, Hampton EM: Toxic carbamazepine concentrations following cardiothoracic surgery and myocardial infarction. DICP Ann Pharmacother 1990;24:822–826.

142 Tetzlaff JE: Intraoperative defect in haemostasis in a child receiving valproic acid. Can J Anaesth 1991;38:222–224.

Krishna DasGupta, MD, Citadel Psychiatric Clinic, 2001 Reed Road,
Fort Wayne, IN 46815 (USA)

Subject Index

Esophageal motility disorder
  globus treatment 49, 50
  psychiatric disorder in patients 49, 50

Fluoxetine
  cardiac effects 35
  depression treatment in cancer patients
    117
  effect of cirrhosis on metabolism 10,
    11
  half-life 10, 11, 117
  mechanism of action 35
  overdose attempts 33, 34
  protein binding 10
  recommendations in disease
    cardiac disease 31, 35
    epilepsy 67
    kidney disease 17
    Parkinson's disease 72
    pulmonary disease 23, 24
  side effects 35, 51
Folliculitis, lithium association 92

Gastritis, psychotropic therapy 50
Gastroparesis, psychotropic therapy 50
Globus, *see* Esophageal motility disorder
Glucose intolerance, mania treatment in
  patients 146

Haloperidol
  delirium treatment in cancer 120, 121
  hepatotoxicity 9, 10, 56
  recommendations in disease
    cardiac disease 40
    epilepsy 63, 64
Hepatorenal syndrome, development in
  liver disease 8, 12
Herpes, lithium treatment 100, 101
Human immunodeficiency virus, *see*
  Acquired immune deficiency syndrome
Huntington's disease
  age of onset 74
  diagnosis 74
  gene locus 74
  psychiatric disorders in patients 75
  psychotropic drug therapy 74, 75
Hypothyroidism, drug induction 139–141

Imipramine, recommendations in cardiac
  disease 31, 32
Immunotherapy, psychiatric disorders in
  patients 123
Infectious diseases, mania treatment 154
Irritable bowel syndrome
  psychiatric disorder in patients 49, 52
  psychotropic therapy 52, 53
  treatment 52, 53

Kidney, *see also* Renal insufficiency
  drug clearance 7
  failure etiology
    intrarenal 13
    postrenal 13
    prerenal 13
  lithium effects 141, 142
  measures of function 14

Leishmaniasis, treatment 101
Leukocytoplastic vasculitis
  induction by antidepressants 97
  lesions 97
Lithium
  cutaneous side effects 90–95, 145
  depression treatment in cancer patients
    116
  excretion 12, 18
  gastrointestinal side effects 51, 54, 147
  herpes simplex treatment 100, 101, 154
  interaction with anesthetics 155
  mania treatment 139–156
  nephrotoxicity 18
  neurotoxicity 150
  recommendations in disease
    calcium disorders 149, 150
    cancer 153
    cardiovascular disease 143, 144
    gastrointestinal disease 147
    glucose intolerance 146
    hematologic disease 152
    infectious diseases 154
    kidney disease 18, 19, 142, 143
    liver disease 148
    neurological disorders 150, 151
    Parkinson's disease 73
    pulmonary disease 146, 147

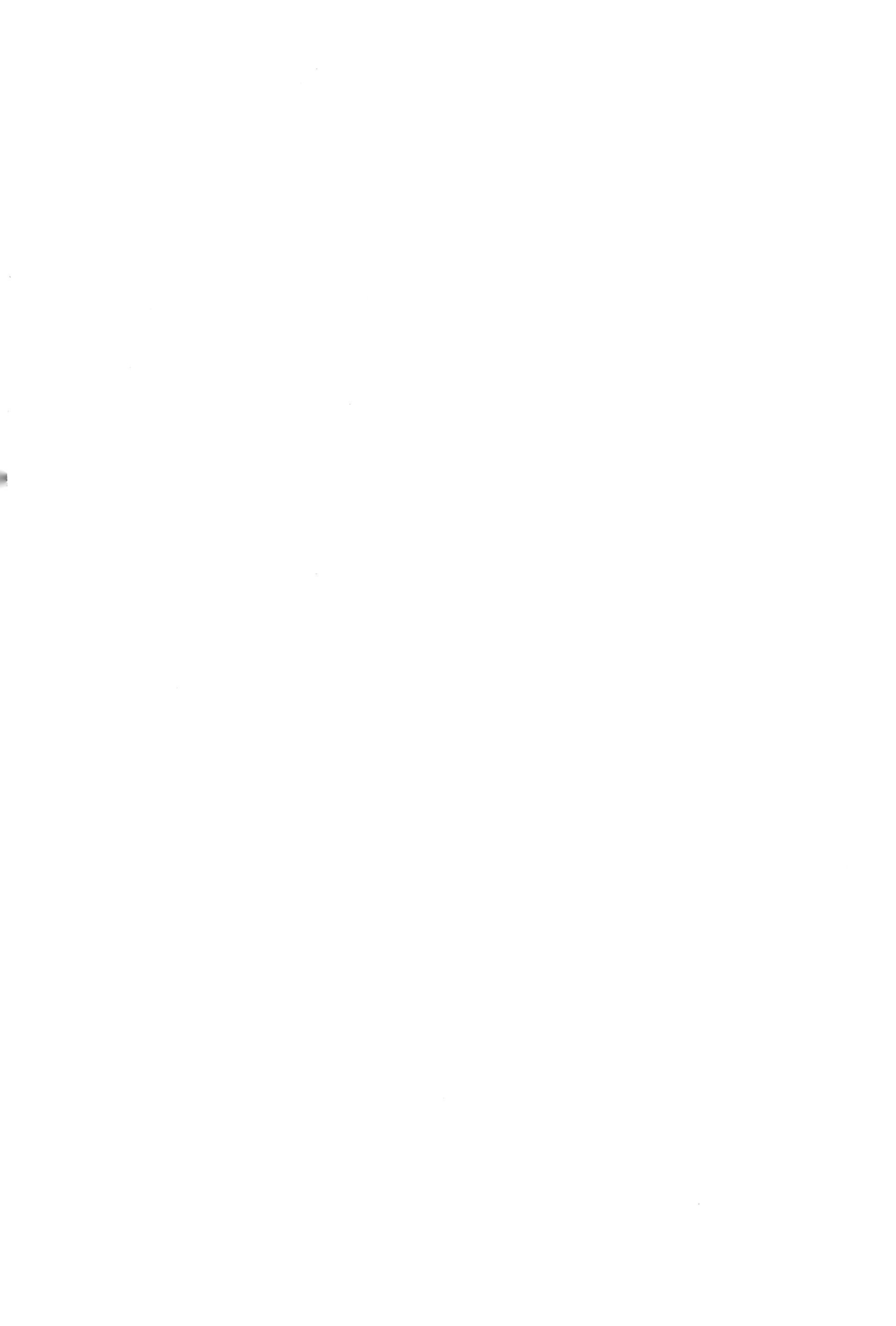